MCQ TUTO

MCQ TUTOR: ANAESTHESIA
Second Edition

A.W. GROGONO, MD, FFARCS
Professor and Chairman, Department of Anesthesiology,
Tulane University School of Medicine, New Orleans

T. HILARY HOWELLS, MB, BS, FFARCS
Director, Department of Anaesthesia,
The Royal Free Hospital, London

J. L. SELTZER, MD
Associate Professor of Anesthesiology, Jefferson Medical College
of Thomas Jefferson University, Philadelphia

and

SUSAN MANN, MD, FFARCS
Senior Registrar, University Hospital, Nottingham

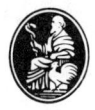

WILLIAM HEINEMANN MEDICAL BOOKS LIMITED
London

First published 1975

Second edition 1983

© A.W. Grogono, T.H. Howells, J.L. Seltzer and S. Mann, 1983

ISBN 0-433-15360-1

Filmset in 10/11pt Compugraphic English Times by
CK Typesetters Ltd., Sutton, Surrey.
Printed and bound in Great Britain by
Redwood Burn Ltd., Trowbridge and Melksham.

CONTENTS

PREFACE

This tutor is a second collection in a series of multiple choice questions which are drawn from the basic sciences associated with anaesthesia. Like the previous edition, and in common with the current postgraduate examinations, the standard form of multiple choice questions is used, consisting of a stem and five responses, of which any number may be correct. Students wishing to use the answer sheets at the end of the book should score one mark for each correctly answered item and lose a mark for each incorrect option selected.

This self-assessment exercise is recommended as an invaluable aid for the student reader. One of the main problems that the student faces in the course of his study is the lack of challenge to his learning. This applies in particular to the person studying in isolation or outside centres of teaching who might otherwise meet the first challenge to his knowledge at the examination itself. The MCQ format is a most useful device for such a challenge and the self-assessment facility provided in this book enables the reader to monitor his learning progress.

Another function of the assessment exercise is to familiarise the reader preparing for examination with the scoring system currently in use and to alert him to the care needed in reading the stem of the question and its answer options. It is suggested that the student allocates two minutes per question for completing the answer section.

Questions are laid out on right-hand pages and answers, together with discussions, are found overleaf. The discussion notes ventilate the core of knowledge relevant to each subject and serve to either reassure the reader or to identify a weakness.

If the questions and answers in this book stimulate the student to study areas he would have otherwise neglected or to review subjects about which his understanding was poor, then the authors will have fulfilled their purpose.

A. W. Grogono, MD, FFARCS
T. Hilary Howells, MB, BS, FFARCS
J. L. Seltzer, MD
Susan Mann, MD, FFARCS

INTRODUCTION

Multiple choice questions are so widely used in all examinations that few anaesthetists will now enter the speciality without having already been exposed to this type of assessment. The reasons for the popularity of MCQs are not difficult to find. Examiners will readily admit that the examination process is fallible. The outcome depends in part on the candidate's knowledge and ability, but will also depend on the examiners' aptitudes in constructing and marking a suitable test. Subjectivity on the part of the examiner can greatly affect the results obtained with the traditional essay paper and *viva voce*. Multiple choice examinations have a much greater degree of objectivity than these traditional alternatives, and are a more reliable method of testing ability. MCQ examinations allow the examiners to test the candidates' factual knowledge over a broad range of the syllabus using a series of tried and reliable questions.

From the examiner's standpoint multiple choice tests do suffer from some limitations. In general they constitute a somewhat superficial test of knowledge. They do not readily allow testing either for originality or the ability to reason and expound an argument. These limitations should be taken into account when considering the strategy you should use in tackling one of these tests.

There are many different types of multiple choice question. The questions in this book are identical in structure to those used in all the MCQ examinations of the Faculty of Anaesthetists. They consist of a stem, in which a problem is posed in the form of a question or statement, and five options, numbered A to E or 1 to 5. The candidate is asked to state in respect of each and every option whether or not it is a correct solution of the problem posed in the stem. Each option may be a true or false solution. This type of item is known as a 'determinate' or 'multiple true–false' type of question. Outside the English Faculty's examinations the 'single correct response' type of question is widely used. This again consists of a stem and five alternative options, but the candidate is told that only one of these options is correct, or that there is a single 'best' answer. Yet another variation on the MCQ theme is the question in which the candidate is given a number of suggested solutions from which to choose. Following the stem and various options, the candidate may then be told to put A if he thinks options 1, 2 and 3 are correct, B if he thinks 1 and 4 are the correct options and so on. This type of question, together with the single correct response type, is used in the examinations of the Australian Faculty of Anaesthetists. The importance of recognising these different types of question is that different methods of marking are used in each, and this must influence your strategy in planning your answers. In assessing multiple true–false types of questions examiners will allot plus marks for correct responses and deduct marks for incorrect answers. You should thus be deterred with this type of question from hazarding wild guesses. With the single correct response, question marks are not usually deducted for an incorrect answer and here, if you are not sure of the correct answer, it is to your advantage to guess—you cannot lose by doing this and may be lucky and gain.

The usual method of marking multiple true–false questions of the type contained in this book is to give one mark for each option answered correctly and deduct a mark for each option incorrectly answered. No marks are added or deducted for options which are not answered. In a question with five options the candidate who answers all correctly will score $+5$ and five incorrect answers will receive a score of -5. In theory, wild guesses should be randomly correct or incorrect and should lead to a score of zero, so that guessing is unlikely to improve your score. Whilst the $+1/-1$ approach is the most commonly used marking method, other schemes have been tried. There is a probably apocryphal story of an examination (not held in the UK) in which, in order more positively to deter guessing the examiners decided to give one mark for correct answers and deduct two marks for incorrect ones. This system had a rapid demise, for it led to the pass mark for the examination being close to zero or even negative. The wise candidates rapidly learned that regardless of factual knowledge the chances of passing the examination were high even if you answered no questions at all, and tended to diminish as you tackled more questions!

How should one tackle an examination made up of questions like those found in this book? As in all examinations an over-riding rule is to read each question carefully. Much thought is always given to the exact wording of multiple choice questions, and every word in the stem and options is there for a reason. Authorities agree that the most efficient way of dealing with a multiple choice test is to go through the paper once and answer those options about which you have little doubt. Having done that you should then read through the question paper again. Although wild guessing is a waste of time, experience has shown that when one is only moderately sure of a correct answer, it is better to follow your hunch than to leave the option unanswered.

Introduction

Always remember that in this type of test time is at a premium. For most MCQ papers the examiners allow two minutes for each total question. If the questions have been well designed you should not have to spend much time trying to work out what the stem means or what the examiners are getting at. Multiple choice questions are not intended to probe deeply into your ability to reason out answers, and if you find yourself doing this you have most probably misunderstood the question. Do not waste time trying to interpret what seems to you to be a difficult or complex question, and do not search deeply for catches. An examiner is usually present throughout the course of a multiple choice examination. Do not hesitate to ask for his assistance if you think there is a severe ambiguity in a question—printing errors do sometimes occur.

MCQ examinations are commonly marked by means of a computer, and you have to give your answers in a way that the computer can interpret. The Faculty of Anaesthetists gives candidates for its MCQ examinations advice as to how to do this. You must use the pencil they provide to fill in the answer cards, fill in the boxes, lozenges or ovals in the way illustrated on the front of the question book, and follow the methods they give for changing any answers. You are advised initially to mark your responses by putting ticks or crosses in the question book and then transcribing these to the answer card or cards. If you have had a great deal of MCQ experience you may feel confident about entering the answers directly. There is an increased danger in doing this that you will put the answers to a question in the space intended for the answers to a different question, and no computer can know that the answers you have given for question 10 are really the answers to question 12.

Candidates taking Fellowship examinations often ask how many MCQ questions they need to answer in order to pass. This is a difficult question to answer. The outcome of an MCQ examination is a mark in the range of -100% to $+100\%$ of the total possible score. Examinations vary in their passmark, but for most of the FFA multiple choice examinations you will pass if you get a mark of $+55$ to $+60\%$. It is, however, most dangerous to think during an examination that because you have now answered enough items to give you a score of say 60%, you can stop. There are three good reasons for not doing this. First, it is very possible that some of your answers are wrong. You cannot know this, otherwise you would have answered differently. Second, many MCQ examinations (for instance the Primary FFA) are subdivided into a number of separate sections that are assessed independently. If you stop before the end of the paper you may score well in some sections but, by virtue of omission, fail badly in others. Third, the actual pass mark usually changes each time an examination is held. MCQ papers inevitably vary as to their overall difficulty. In order to compensate for this the pass mark is commonly adjusted using the candidates' performance in so-called discriminator questions which have been used in previous examinations. If, for instance, the overall scores in a MCQ test are lower than the previous time it was taken but the results in repeated discriminator questions are the same as previously, the pass mark will be adjusted downwards to allow the same proportion of candidates through. A better or a worse performance than previously is interpreted by the examiners as evidence of overall higher or lower standards in the candidates sitting the examination and will also result in adjustment of the pass mark.

A corollary of this is that the impression that in any examination a multiple choice paper is easier or harder than last time is illusory. A paper that appears harder may in fact be easier to pass, and conversely (and much more dangerous if you relax your standards) an apparently easy paper usually demands a greater number of correct answers if you are to achieve success.

So far in this introduction we have concentrated upon the place of the multiple choice question in the examination context. This book, however, is not an examination. Its intent is to allow you to use the MCQs it contains for self-test, to practise your ability to answer such questions and by means of the commentary on each question to improve and broaden your knowledge of the subject matter the questions cover. Because, with this book, you do not lose marks for wrong answers it is important, when using these questions to test your ability, that you conscientiously put down an answer for each option in each question. In this way you will learn of the gaps in your knowledge and painlessly gain information.

Professor C. M. Conway
Westminster Hospital, London
1983

1. PHARMACOLOGY

1.1. Drug receptors:

    A. Are theoretical structures created to help explain the action of drugs
    B. React with drugs to produce the pharmacologic effect
    C. Are stimulated by agonists
    D. Are blocked by antagonists
    E. Can be both stimulated and blocked by the same drug.

1.2. Drugs cross cell membranes by:

    A. Diffusion
    B. Lipolysis
    C. Penetration
    D. Active transport
    E. Ionization.

1.3. Protein binding of drugs:

    A. Is entirely due to van der Waal forces
    B. Is dependent upon the concentration of the drug
    C. May be decreased in liver disease
    D. May be reduced by other drugs occupying the same sites
    E. Is clinically insignificant.

Answers overleaf

1.1. B, C, D, E

Drug receptors are actual physical or molecular sites on cell membranes where the drugs produce their pharmacological effects. Agonists stimulate receptors while antagonists block them. Some drugs can have both agonist and antagonist properties.

1.2. A, C, D.

The non-ionized form of a drug is lipid soluble and passes through membranes. The ratio between dissociated and undissociated forms of a drug depends upon the pH of the medium and the pK of the drug.

Penetration occurs through pores in membranes. This is a slow process and no energy is required.

Active transport requires energy. It is thought to involve an intermediate carrier which binds the drug on one side of the membrane and releases the drug on the other side. Some drugs work by inhibiting this active transport process.

1.3. B, C, D

Many drugs are bound to plasma proteins (both albumin and globulin). The amount of binding is dependent on the concentration of the drug in the plasma. Many binding forces are probably involved, such as van der Waal forces and ionic bonding.

Low circulating albumin secondary to liver disease, or the presence of other drugs on the binding sites, will decrease the amount of bound drug thus allowing more unbound drug to exert a greater effect than expected. This exaggerated response can be clinically significant. Protein binding also occurs at cellular level.

1.4. Factors that determine the concentration of a drug at its site of action include:

A. The biochemical effect of the drug
B. The rate of absorption
C. The distribution of the drug
D. The biotransformation of the drug
E. The excretion of the drug.

1.5. The MAC of an inhalational anaesthetic agent:

A. Is the maximal allowable concentration that can be given
B. Must be determined in unpremedicated subjects
C. Is determined by measuring the inspired concentration of an agent
D. Indicates when 50% of the population will not move when a surgical incision is made
E. Is used to indicate equipotent concentrations of inhalational agents.

1.6. The major biochemical processes by which drugs are metabolized include:

A. Oxidation
B. Reduction
C. Hydrolysis
D. Spontaneous degeneration
E. Conjugation.

Answers overleaf

1.4. B, C, D, E

Pharmacokinetics is concerned with: (1) absorption, (2) distribution, (3) biotransformation, (4) binding to tissues and (5) excretion of drugs. These five factors, plus the dosage of the drug, determine the concentration at its site of action.

Pharmacodynamics is concerned with the biochemical and physiological effects of drugs, as well as their mechanisms of action.

1.5. B, D, E

MAC signifies the 'minimal alveolar concentration' of an inhalational agent that prevents movement in 50% of a population when a surgical stimulation (incision) is applied. It is determined by measuring the end expiratory concentration of the agent. Only the agent for which the MAC is being determined is administered. The subjects are unpremedicated and do not receive N_2O or muscle relaxants.

A one MAC concentration of any agent is equipotent, although the actual percentage of the agents being delivered is different (1 MAC halothane is 0.77% while 1 MAC enflurane is 1.68%; therefore 1.68% of enflurane is equipotent to 0.77% of halothane).

1.6. A, B, C, E

Oxidation reactions include hydroxylation, dealkylation, deamination, and sulphoxide formation. Reduction reactions occur in the metabolism of a small number of drugs only. Many drugs, especially esters, used in anaesthesia are deactivated by hydrolysis. Conjugation occurs in the liver forming sulphates and glucuronides.

1.7. Epileptic activity:

A. Is frequently noted on electroencephalography (EEG) with one MAC halothane anaesthesia
B. Is more likely to appear under enflurane anaesthesia if the patient is hypoventilated
C. Under enflurane anaesthesia may be manifested by facial twitching
D. On EEG may continue for 6–30 days after deep enflurane anaesthesia
E. Is abolished under enflurane anaesthesia by increasing the inspired concentration and hyperventilating the patient.

1.8. Enflurane:

A. Increases cerebral metabolism
B. Causes cerebral vasodilation
C. Decreases intracranial pressure
D. Increases cerebral oxygen consumption
E. Does not affect cerebral blood flow.

1.9. Nitrous oxide (N_2O)

A. Increases cardiac output
B. Decreases peripheral resistance
C. Causes no significant changes in arterial blood pressure
D. Increases heart rate
E. Sensitises the heart to exogenous catecholamines.

1.10. Halothane:

A. Increases gastrointestinal tract motility
B. Increases cerebral blood flow
C. Raises intracranial pressure
D. Increases cerebral metabolism
E. Causes cerebral vasoconstriction in the presence of hyperventilation.

Answers overleaf

1.7. C, D

Of the commonly used inhalational agents only enflurane produces epileptic activity. It appears on EEG at higher concentration (usually over 3%) especially when the patient is hyperventilated. Reduction of the inspired concentration and avoidance of hyperventilation will abolish the overt manifestation of the epileptic activity (facial twitching and limb movement). However, after prolonged deep enflurane anaesthesia, EEG changes may persist for 6–30 days.

1.8. B

Enflurane decreases cerebral oxygen consumption and metabolism. Cerebral vasodilation takes place; if the mean arterial pressure is constant the blood flow increases, if the arterial pressure falls blood flow may stay constant or fall. Intracranial pressure usually increases.

1.9. C

N_2O decreases cardiac output and increases peripheral vascular resistance. The two changes balance each other and therefore no change in arterial blood pressure occurs. The heart rate usually decreases slightly. The heart is not sensitized to catecholamines by N_2O.

1.10. B, C

Halothane causes neither salivation nor gastric secretion, and gut motility is depressed. It causes cerebral vasodilation, thus increasing blood flow and tending to cause a rise in intracranial pressure. Prior hyperventilation modifies, but does not completely prevent, the cerebral vasodilation and intracranial pressure rise associated with halothane administration.

Pharmacology

1.11. Halothane causes:

    A. Inhibition of the effects of the sympathetic nervous system on the cardiovascular system
    B. Central vasomotor depression
    C. Direct myocardial depression
    D. An increase in systemic vascular resistance
    E. Stimulation of the baroreceptors.

1.12. Cardiac dysrhythmias during inhalational anaesthesia:

    A. Will occur at 10.9 μg/kg of adrenaline if enflurane is the agent being used
    B. Will occur at 2.1 μg/kg of adrenaline if halothane is the agent being used
    C. Are less frequent during light anaesthesia and moderate hypercarbia
    D. May result from the depression of ventricular automaticity associated with inhalation of halogenated hydrocarbons
    E. Are less likely to occur with halothane because it has no effect on ventricular conduction time.

1.13. Enflurane anaesthesia:

    A. Increases systemic vascular resistance
    B. Decreases cardiac output
    C. Causes about a 20% decrease in heart rate
    D. Increases mean arterial pressure
    E. Affects haemodynamics mainly through the vasomotor centre.

1.14. Respiratory depression associated with inhalational anaesthetics:

    A. Is greater with halothane than enflurane
    B. Is partially caused by a slowing of the respiratory rate
    C. May limit the depth of anaesthesia that can be achieved with spontaneous breathing
    D. Causes reduced responses to both hypoxia and hypercarbia
    E. Is partially due to a decreased tidal volume.

Answers overleaf

1.11. A, B, C

There is a dose-related fall in arterial blood pressure associated with halothane anaesthesia. This causes decreased sympathetic activity, central vasomotor depression, and probable depression of the baroreceptors. Myocardial contractility is depressed and there is a slight fall in systemic vascular resistance.

1.12. A, B, D

Enflurane is much more compatible with adrenaline than either halothane or isoflurane, with which dysrhythmias develop at 6.7 μg/kg adrenaline. Light anaesthesia and hypercarbia increase endogenous catecholamine levels and further predispose to dysrhythmias. Halogenated hydrocarbons generally decrease the heart rate and ventricular automaticity which probably predisposes to dysrhythmia. Halothane may be more dysrhythmogenic than enflurane because while both prolong A–V conduction halothane also depresses ventricular conduction time.

1.13. B

Enflurane directly depresses myocardial contractility, thus reducing cardiac output. Its effect on pulse rate varies. If the heart rate is rapid pre-induction it may slow. In other studies a tachycardia has been reported. The systemic vascular resistance is usually decreased and thus coupled with the fall in cardiac output the mean arterial pressure falls.

1.14. C, D, E

Enflurane causes greater respiratory depression than halothane in rats, dogs and man. In general, inhalational agents decrease the tidal volume and increase the respiratory rate (an exception is diethyl ether which initially causes an increased tidal volume but, at deeper levels of anaesthesia, is also a respiratory depressant). With agents that cause marked respiratory depression it may be impossible to reach deeper levels of anaesthesia because apnoea occurs first.

1.15. Muscle relaxation provided by enflurane:

    A. Is a result of actions on the motor cortex
    B. Is a result of actions at the myoneural junction
    C. May be sufficient for abdominal surgery
    D. Antagonizes non-depolarizing neuromuscular relaxants
    E. Is dose-dependent.

1.16. Enflurane:

    A. Is an ether
    B. Is inflammable but not explosive in concentrations over 5%
    C. Has the structural formula:

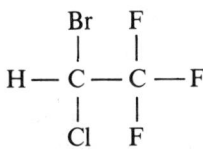

    D. Is metabolized to yield free bromide ions
    E. Is metabolized to yield free fluoride ions.

1.17. Nitrous oxide (N_2O):

    A. Decreases the respiratory response to hypercarbia
    B. Is slightly less soluble than N_2
    C. May be associated with postoperative hearing loss
    D. Has been associated with bone marrow aplasia after prolonged administration
    E. Does not support combustion.

Answers overleaf

1.15. B, C, E

Dose-dependent blockade of neuromuscular transmission occurs with enflurane. It is most likely due to direct effects at the neuromuscular junction. Non-depolarizing neuromuscular blocking agents are potentiated by enflurane. Deep enflurane anaesthesia can provide adequate relaxation for abdominal surgery. However, concomitant cardiovascular depression must be accepted.

1.16. A, E

Enflurane has the structural formula:

$$
\begin{array}{ccccccc}
 & \text{Cl} & & \text{F} & & & \text{F} \\
 & | & & | & & & | \\
\text{H} - & \text{C} & - & \text{C} & - \text{O} - & \text{C} & - \text{H} \\
 & | & & | & & & | \\
 & \text{F} & & \text{F} & & & \text{F}
\end{array}
$$

It is an ether and is both non-flammable and non-explosive when mixed with oxygen throughout the entire clinical range.

Free fluoride ions are metabolic by-products; the maximum fluoride levels are about 25–35 mmol/l, which is below the 50 mmol/l concentration traditionally felt to be necessary for the development of renal dysfunction. However, in patients with known renal disease, enflurane should probably be avoided.

1.17. A, C, D

Nitrous oxide is a gas which has analgesic properties but is a very poor anaesthetic agent when used by itself. It has a slight depressant effect on the response to hypercarbia.

It is 35 times more soluble than N_2, therefore large quantities are available to enter a cavity containing air, making that cavity's volume much larger (i.e. pneumothorax or air in the gut or the middle ear). This diffusion into, and then out of, the middle ear may cause postoperative hearing loss. If the patient breathes air at the end of a nitrous oxide anaesthetic the N_2O comes out of the blood into the lung more rapidly than the N_2 of air enters the blood. This causes the O_2 in the alveoli to be diluted, possibly to hypoxic levels. Bone marrow depression occurs after prolonged administration (several days). N_2O will support combustion and explosions.

1.18. Halothane:

   A. Is mostly eliminated by exhalation
   B. Is partially metabolized in the liver
   C. Is mostly excreted unchanged in the urine
   D. Is metabolized to yield free bromide ions
   E. Is metabolized to trifluracetic acid.

1.19. Midazolam:

   A. Is a β-adrenergic blocker
   B. Has anticonvulsant activity
   C. Produces marked dose-related depression of cardiac output
   D. Does not release histamine
   E. Has a half-life in man of about 2 hours.

1.20. Ketamine:

   A. Has marked analgesic properties
   B. Causes a fall in cardiac output
   C. Increases heart rate
   D. Usually preserves pharyngeal and tracheal reflexes
   E. May cause unpleasant dreams, especially in children.

1.21. Thiopentone:

   A. Has no effect on myocardial contractility
   B. Decreases heart rate
   C. Causes vasodilation
   D. In induction doses of 4 mg/kg lowers blood pressure about 20% in healthy subjects
   E. May have its cardiovascular side effects modified by using small incremental doses.

Answers overleaf

1.18. A, B, D, E

While the major proportion of halothane is eliminated by exhalation, about 12% is metabolized in the liver and the products excreted in the urine. Metabolic products include trifluracetic acid, chloride and bromide ions. Bromide has been associated with prolonged sedation following halothane anaesthesia.

1.19. B, D, E

Midazolam is a water-soluble benzodiazepine and has the advantage over diazepam of not irritating tissues. It exhibits dose-related central nervous system depression and has anticonvulsant activity like diazepam. It does not affect neuromuscular transmission nor does it enhance the effects of neuromuscular blocking agents. It has very mild cardiovascular effects and does not release histamine. Over 95% of the drug is bound to plasma protein and its half-life is thought to be about 2 hours.

1.20. A, C, D

Ketamine is an agent with marked analgesic effects which persist after recovery of consciousness. There is an increase in heart rate, cardiac output and blood pressure associated with catecholamine release. Respiratory and upper airway reflexes are usually maintained, however this cannot be relied upon. The major difficulties associated with its use are prolonged postoperative somnolence following repeated doses and unpleasant dreams in about 6% of adults, but children seem immune.

1.21. C, D

Thiopentone decreases myocardial contractility and causes vasodilation. The heart rate increases with induction doses. In a healthy patient the blood pressure falls approximately 20%. It has recently been shown that giving thiopentone in 50 mg increments every 30 seconds did not significantly modify its cardiovascular effects when compared with a 4 mg/kg dose in healthy adults. High risk patients, such as those who are hypovolaemic or in heart failure, should be given reduced doses (1–3 mg/kg).

1.22. Thiopentone:

A. In 2.5% solution has a pH of about 11
B. Is scarcely metabolized
C. Is an oxybarbiturate
D. Is stable for less than 24 hours after preparation as a solution
E. Is used in 10% solutions.

1.23. Thiopentone:

A. Stimulates the respiratory centre of the brain
B. Alters the patient's response to CO_2
C. Does not depress laryngeal reflexes until deep levels of anaesthesia are reached
D. Usually reduces the depth of respiration
E. Causes bronchospasm in patients with asthma.

1.24. Thiopentone:

A. Causes dose-dependent, progressive depression of the central nervous system
B. Increases cerebral oxygen consumption
C. Causes cerebral vasodilation
D. Increases cerebral blood flow
E. Causes dose-dependent increases in intracranial pressure.

1.25. Suxamethonium:

A. Acts as an antagonist at the neuromuscular junction
B. Is metabolized by hydrolysis in 3–5 minutes
C. Lowers the transmembrane resting potential at the neuromuscular junction
D. Acts by allowing shift of sodium and potassium ions
E. Is antagonistic to tubocurarine.

Answers overleaf

1.22. A

Thiopentone is a relatively stable, ultra-short-acting barbiturate which is almost completely metabolized in the liver. It is the sulphur analogue of pentobarbitone and is therefore a thiobarbiturate. The solution is very alkaline, but remains stable for days after it is prepared. Commonly used solutions are 2 or 2.5%. Solutions of 5 and 10% can be irritant to tissues especially if extravascular or intra-arterial injection occurs.

1.23. B, C, D

Thiopentone depress the respiratory centre in the brain, changing its response to CO_2. The amount of depression increases with the dose and speed of injection. It takes large doses to depress laryngeal and bronchial reflexes, and stimulation under light thiopentone anaesthesia can cause laryngospasm or bronchospasm. The agent by itself does not cause bronchospasm even in patients with irritable airways.

1.24. A

The cerebral depressant activity of thiopentone progresses as the injected dose increases. Cerebral oxygen consumption, blood flow and intracranial pressure all decrease, making it an ideal agent for intracranial surgery. It has marked anticonvulsive properties and can be used to treat seizures.

1.25. B, C, D, E

Suxamethonium is a depolarizing neuromuscular blocking agent. It acts as an agonist and allows ionic shifts to take place, lowering the resting potential of the membrane. This prevents acetylcholine from acting to effect neuromuscular transmission.

Its action is terminated by hydrolysis in about 3–5 minutes in normal patients. The administration of suxamethonium to a partially curarized patient will antagonize the effect of curare.

1.26. A depolarization block shows the following characteristics:

    A. Fasciculations
    B. First noticeable effect is on the diaphragm
    C. Fade on tetanic stimulation
    D. Lack of post-tetanic facilitation
    E. Reversal with anticholineserase drugs.

1.27. Fasciculations following suxamethonium:

    A. Increase intragastric pressure
    B. Cause postoperative myalgia
    C. Decrease intracranial pressure
    D. Do not change intraocular pressure
    E. Raise the serum potassium levels unless curare is given first.

1.28. A 'dual block' after suxamethonium:

    A. Has depolarizing characteristics
    B. Has non-depolarizing characteristics
    C. Is often of brief duration
    D. Shows some degree of post-tetanic facilitation
    E. May be partially reversed with anticholinesterases.

Answers overleaf

1.26. A, D

Depolarization neuromuscular block (as seen with suxamethonium) progressively affects the muscle of the face, then extremities, trunk and lastly the diaphragm. Because of the depolarization, fasciculation of the muscles are seen. There is no fade of the response to tetanic stimulation and no post-tetanic facilitation of twitch, as seen with curare. A pure depolarization block does not reverse with anticholinesterases and probably will become more intense.

1.27. A, B

Because of fasciculation following suxamethonium, intragastric, intracranial and intraocular pressures rise. Generalized postoperative muscle pain (myalgia) is seen very often in patients who received suxamethonium regardless of degree of fasciculation.

Fasciculations can be markedly reduced by giving a small dose of non-depolarizing neuromuscular blocking agent about 3 minutes before suxamethonium (i.e. 40 μg/kg curare). This does not prevent the rise in serum potassium level, which is the result of depolarization and not the visible fasciculations.

1.28. All correct

A dual block associated with suxamethonium has the characteristics of both a depolarizing and non-depolarizing block. It may first be noticed after 5–10 minutes of an infusion, but will then terminate rapidly. The non-depolarizing characteristics may become prominent after longer periods of administration (usually more than 1–1.5 g over 1 hour periods).

Anticholinesterases will improve the non-depolarizing element of the block, but will potentiate the depolarizing element. Clinically it is best to ventilate the patient until the block wears off, rather than attempting pharmacological reversal.

1.29. Marked hyperkalaemia following administration of suxamethonium may:

A. Occur in patients with upper motor neurone lesions
B. Occur in patients with renal failure
C. Occur in patients who have suffered trauma to skeletal muscle
D. Result in cardiac arrest
E. Be satisfactorily prevented by administering the suxamethonium slowly.

1.30. Which of the following are true about receptors in the sympathetic nervous system?

A. Stimulation of β_1 receptors increases the rate, automaticity and contractility of the heart
B. Vascular resistance is inceased by β_2 stimulation
C. Airway resistance is increased by β_2 stimulation
D. Renal vascular resistance is increased by α stimulation
E. Renal vascular resistance is decreased by dopaminergic stimulation.

1.31. Adrenaline administered to adults:

A. At the rate of 1-2 μg/min will have primarily α effects
B. At the rate of 2-10 μg/min will have both α and β effects
C. May cause tachycardia and dysrhythmias
D. May cause metabolic acidosis
E. Is the drug of choice for hypotension following a myocardial infarction.

Answers overleaf

1.29. A, C, D

The following conditions have been associated with hyperkalaemia following suxamethonium: burns, muscle trauma, upper and lower motor neurone lesions and some muscle diseases. The susceptibility continues until healing of the injury, or the active stage of the disease, passes.

Slow administration of suxamethonium can not be relied upon to prevent the hyperkalaemic response. Therefore, suxamethonium is best avoided in susceptible patients.

Renal failure patients show the normal increase in serum potassium following suxamethonium (0.5 mmol/1). Therefore if their potassium levels are normal pre-induction, they should not become hyperkalaemic.

1.30. A, D, E

It is generally accepted that there are four distinct receptor sites in the sympathetic nervous system; α, β_1, β_2, and dopaminergic. β_1 is confined to the heart, increasing rate, automaticity and contractility; β_2 stimulation decreases vascular and airway resistance; α stimulation causes vascular constriction, and this includes the renal artery. However, dopaminergic stimulation dilates the renal artery.

1.31. B, C, D

The effect of adrenaline varies with its rate of administration. When given to the average adult, $1-2$ μg/min has β effects, $2-10$ μg/min has both α and β effects and $10-20$ μg/min have α effects. Disadvantages include tachycardia and dysrhythmias, which can be treated with lignocaine. The α effects cause vasoconstriction, which can cause renal failure and/or metabolic acidosis. Unwanted α effects can be treated by using a vasodilator. When used after myocardial infarction its positive inotropic effect and tachycardia may extend the infarct.

1.32. Which of the following are true?

A. Dobutamine dilates the renal artery
B. Ephedrine decreases systemic vascular resistance
C. Methoxamine increases cardiac output
D. Phenylephrine is a pure β drug
E. Dobutamine causes more tachycardia than dopamine.

1.33. Sodium nitroprusside administration:

A. Causes venous vasodilation with little effect on the arterial vessels
B. Decreases cardiac output
C. Has a direct action on the vascular smooth muscle
D. May cause a fall in Pao_2
E. Has not been associated with any significant side effects.

1.34. Intravenous nitroglycerine:

A. Increases venous capacitance
B. Decrease the heart size and wall tension
C. Is more potent than nitroprusside in controlling arterial hypertension
D. May redistribute coronary blood flow to ischaemic myocardium
E. May cause cyanide toxicity.

Answers overleaf

1.32. None

Dobutamine is a positive inotropic agent that causes less tachycardia and dysrhythmia than dopamine. It causes vasodilation mostly in the skeletal muscle and tends to shift blood flow away from the kidney. Ephedrine has both α and β effects, and it increases cardiac output and systemic vascular resistance. Both methoxamine and phenylephrine are almost pure α drugs whose primary effect is vasoconstriction.

1.33. C, D

Sodium nitroprusside is a potent dilator of both arterial and venous vessels acting directly on vascular smooth muscle. By reducing the resistance against which the heart must empty, it increases cardiac output and decreases myocardial oxygen consumption. Where it is being used to treat hypertension, or induce hypotension, the PaO_2 may fall because nitroprusside blocks the pulmonary hypoxic vasoconstriction reflex.

Since cyanide is a metabolic byproduct, the potential of toxicity exists. This may be seen as the development of metabolic acidosis, tachyphylaxis to the drug and a narrowing of the arterial to mixed venous oxygen tensions. It is recommended to limit doses given in long-term therapy to 0.5–1 mg/kg/day, and in short-term therapy to 1.5 mg/kg/day in order to avoid cyanide toxicity.

1.34. A, B, D

Intravenous preparations of nitroglycerine have a greater effect on venous circulation than the arterial. The preload of the heart is reduced. Its effect on arterial hypertension is much less than that of nitroprusside. However it seems to have the advantage of improving myocardial oxygenation during ischaemia. Although the development of methaemoglobinaemia is a theoretical possibility, it has not been reported. There is no cyanide toxicity with nitroglycerine.

1.35. Atropine:

- **A.** Completely blocks the vagus nerve in doses of 0.4 mg/70 kg
- **B.** In very low doses may cause bradycardia
- **C.** Increases physiological dead space
- **D.** Produces moderate central nervous depression
- **E.** Dilates the pupil of the eye following premedicant dosage.

1.36. Hyoscine, when compared with atropine:

- **A.** Has greater sedative effects
- **B.** Has less antisialogogue effect
- **C.** Has greater antiemetic effect
- **D.** Produces a greater amount of tachycardia
- **E.** Is more likely to produce confusion in the elderly.

1.37. Isoprenaline:

- **A.** Stimulates the baroreceptors to cause bradycardia
- **B.** Is the drug of choice for bronchospasm
- **C.** Is used in 1-5 μg/min doses to produce positive inotropic activity in adults
- **D.** Is the drug of choice in complete heart block
- **E.** May cause hypotension.

1.38. Dopamine:

- **A.** Stimulates cardiac output
- **B.** May vasodilate
- **C.** May vasoconstrict
- **D.** In high doses has all the side effects of adrenaline
- **E.** Is more potent than adrenaline or isoprenaline.

Answers overleaf

1.35. B, C

Atropine is a belladonna alkaloid which is generally used in anaesthesia to prevent or treat bradycardia and to inhibit secretions. To completely block the cardiac vagus, 2–3 mg must be given to the average adult. Very small doses may cause a bradycardia secondary to stimulation of the vagal nucleus in the medulla. Anatomical and, therefore, physiological dead space is increased because of bronchial dilation. In clinical doses 0.4–0.6 mg/70 kg there is little CNS effect. While larger systemic doses of atropine will dilate the pupil, conventional pre-operative doses given intramuscularly have little ocular effect.

1.36. A, C, E

Hyoscine has greater sedative, antisialogogue and antiemetic effects. It produces less vagal blockade to the heart and is therefore not the treatment of choice for reflex bradycardias. In the old and very young it may produce restlessness and confusion.

1.37. C, D, E

Isoprenaline's effect is almost entirely β-adrenergic. It does not stimulate the baroreceptors and therefore increases heart rate due to its β effect. It may cause tachycardia and dysrhythmias. Due to its β_2 effect, it dilates peripheral vessels and can cause hypotension. The usual adult dose for positive inotropic effect is 1-5 μg/min. It is very effective in increasing ventricular rate in complete heart block until a pacemaker is available. There are better drugs, which only have β_2 effects (i.e. terbutaline), available for the treatment of bronchospasm.

1.38. A, B, C, D

There are coronary, renal and mesenteric dopaminergic receptors. In low doses of 2 μg/kg, only the dopaminergic receptors are stimulated. This stimulation causes vasodilation of the mesenteric and renal arteries. Some vasodilation persists up to doses of 20 μg/kg. In doses up to 10 μg/kg there will be an increased cardiac output with vasodilation that shifts blood flow to 'vital organs' (kidneys). At doses above 20 μg/kg all the unwanted side effects of vasoconstriction, seen with adrenaline, appear.

1.39. Glucagon:

   A. Has negative inotropic effects
   B. May cause tachycardia
   C. Has its own independent receptor sites in the heart
   D. Potentiates propranolol
   E. Should be given as a 3–10 mg bolus followed by a 70 μg/kg/min infusion.

1.40. Lignocaine

   A. Stabilizes the membranes of excitable cells
   B. Produces a tachycardia
   C. Decreases cardiac output
   D. Is useful in treating ventricular dysrhythmia
   E. May improve conduction through the A-V node.

1.41. Propranolol:

   A. Is effective in treating heart block
   B. Increases cardiac output
   C. May cause bronchospasm
   D. Is given in incremental intravenous doses of 40 mg
   E. Has α blocking properties.

Answers overleaf

1.39. B, C, E

Glucagon stimulates cardiac activity by acting at receptor sites in the heart that are independent of the sympathetic nervous system. Because of its independent site of action it has been used as an antagonist to myocardial depression due to β blockade. It may cause tachycardia. Administration is as mentioned in answer E.

1.40. A, D, E

Lignocaine stabilizes membranes of excitable cells and is usually the drug of choice for treating acute ventricular dysrhythmias. In standard doses it does not change the heart rate or affect myocardial contractility. It is not useful for supraventricular dysrhythmias and may actually make them worse by enhancing A–V conduction, thus accentuating the ventricular response.

1.41. C

Propranolol is a β-adrenergic blocker. It blocks both β_1 and β_2 activity. New drugs in this class are more selective in their activity. It slows conduction through the heart. Cardiac output decreases and β_2 blockade may cause broncohspasm. Oral doses are much higher than intravenous ones because after absorption from the gut the drug passes through the liver where a great deal of it is inactivated. When given intravenously, 0.2–1 mg increments should be used with a maximum dose of about 5 mg.

1.42. Calcium chloride:

A. Is physiologically active in the un-ionized state
B. Increases the systemic vascular resistance
C. May cause ventricular irritability
D. Potentiates the actions of potassium
E. Increases stroke volume.

1.43. Tricyclic antidepressants:

A. Work by depressing the formation of noradrenaline in the central nervous system
B. May cause hypertension
C. May cause arrhythmias and congestive heart failure
D. Have been associated with renal failure
E. May produce sedation.

1.44. Benzodiazepines:

A. Produce generalized depression of the central nervous system
B. Have mainly antidepressant activity
C. Are potent respiratory depressants
D. Produce minor degrees of cardiovascular depression
E. Have an anticonvulsant effect.

Answers overleaf

Pharmacology

1.42. B, C, E

Ionized calcium is the active form. Its cardiovascular effects include an increase in stroke volume, $\delta p/\delta t$ and systemic vascular resistance; with a decrease in heart rate, left ventricular end diastolic pressure. The overall effect is usually an increase in blood pressure. $CaCl_2$ is useful in antagonizing the myocardial depressive effects of inhalational anaesthetics. ECG changes associated with $CaCl_2$ administration include a shortening of the QT interval without changes in the T wave. High blood levels may cause ventricular irritability, especially in the presence of digitalization or low potassium levels. Calcium and potassium are antagonistic to each other. The usual dose of $CaCl_2$ for positive inotropic effects is 3–7 mg/kg. The action last 15–30 minutes.

1.43. B, C, E

Depression is the most common adult psychiatric condition and the tricyclic antidepressants are the most popular therapeutic agents. They work by preventing the reuptake of noradrenaline by sympathetic nerves. Their use is associated with both hypertension and postural hypotension. Tachycardia, palpitations, arrhythmias and congestive heart failure have been associated with their use. ECG changes noted include flattened T-waves and prolonged A–V conduction. They also produce sedation. Adverse effects include dry mouth, constipation and blurred vision. Both bone marrow depression and cholestatic jaundice have been reported in conjuction with their use.

1.44. D, E

The benzodiazepines include such drugs as chlordiazepoxide (Librium), diazepam (Valium), oxazepam (Serax), and flurazepam (Dalmane). They are sedative, anti-anxiety drugs and work relatively selectively on the limbic system. Even in large doses they produce little respiratory or cardiovascular depression. They produce skeletal muscle relaxation, the mode and site of which are not known. The anticonvulsant effects prevent propagation of potentials and generalization of seizures originating from a focus but do not seem to depress the focus itself.

1.45. Butyrophenones:

   A. Have an antiemetic effect which lasts as long as 7 hours
   B. Cause tachypnoea
   C. Have α-adrenergic blocking properties
   D. Sensitize the heart to adrenaline induced dysrhythmias
   E. May cause extrapyramidal effects.

1.46. Antihistamines:

   A. Prevent the liberation of histamine from mast cells
   B. Are competitive antagonists of histamine
   C. Are used in allergic reactions to reverse the effects of histamine
   D. Have local anaesthetic properties
   E. Have sympathomimetic activity.

Answers overleaf

1.45. A, C, E

Droperidol is a butyrophenone used in neuroleptic anaesthesia. These drugs are strong antiemetics which produce sedation. The respiratory rate drops slightly with an increase in tidal volume. They are mild α-blockers. The threshold for adrenaline induced dysrhythmia is increased by about 75%. Extrapyramidal effects can be a problem with butyrophenones. They consist of muscle tremor, dystonia and Parkinson-like movements.

1.46. B, D

Antihistimines are competitive antagontists of histamine. They prevent histamine from acting on its effector organs, but do not prevent its liberation. Used for allergic reactions they block further effects of histamine, but do not reverse damage that has occurred. Adrenaline is the physiological antagonist of histamine. Most antihistamines have local anaesthetic properties; many have quinidine-like effects on the heart and, like atropine, have parasympatholytic actions; most produce sedation.

2. PHYSIOLOGY

2.1. Which of the following are true?

A. The oxyhaemoglobin dissociation curve is nearly linear
B. With a PaO_2 = 100 mmHg, 100 ml of blood holds 0.3 ml of O_2 in solution
C. One gram of haemoglobin can hold 20 ml of O_2
D. The normal adult consumes 250 ml of O_2 per minute
E. At a PaO_2 of 40 mmHg the haemoglobin is about 40% saturated.

2.2. The difference between alveolar oxygen partial pressure and arterial oxygen partial pressure (A-aDO$_2$)

A. Is increased by a higher FIO_2
B. Is not affected by true shunt
C. Is increased by lowering the V/Q ratio
D. Should completely disappear if 100% O_2 is breathed
E. Is increased by lowering the mixed venous oxygen partial pressure.

2.3. The closing volume of the lung:

A. Is the lung volume at which all alveoli are closed
B. Increases when a subject lies down
C. Decreases when a subject lies down
D. Is measured by the single breath nitrogen test
E. Is always greater than the residual volume

Answers overleaf

2.1. B, D

The oxyhaemoglobin dissociation curve is 'S' shaped. The upper knee of the curve is at about 70% saturation, which corresponds to a PaO_2 of 40 mmHg. Below this point on the curve, small changes in PaO_2 are associated with large changes in saturation. One gram of haemoglobin when fully saturated carries 1.39 ml of O_2. Therefore, 100 ml of blood with a haemoglobin concentration of 15 g/100 ml can carry about 20 ml of O_2 ($15 \times 1.39 = 20.85$ ml/100 ml blood).

2.2. A, C, E

The alveolar–arterial PO_2 difference (A-aDO$_2$) is normally 5 to 25 mmHg, increasing with the patient's age. It will be increased by (1) a raised FIo_2; (2) venous admixture (either low V/Q or true shunt), or (3) low $P\bar{v}o_2$.

2.3. D

The closing volume is measured by observing the nitrogen concentration during exhalation following a single oxygen breath. The point at which the concentration tends to rise is taken as representing the point where airways at the base of the lung are beginning to close (the ones which opened last and received the pure oxygen in contrast with those already open and filled with air). Lying down does not change the volume at which closure occurs; it does reduce the volume of the lungs and tends therefore to cause the lungs to operate within the closing volume, thus enhancing shunting. The closing volume is not always greater than the residual volume. Some teenagers can maximally exhale without closing airways.

2.4. Which of the following are true?

A. Maximum breathing capacity shows how effective bronchodilators may be for a given patient

B. FEV_1 is that part of a forced vital capacity that can be exhaled in one minute

C. The lower limit of normal for the FEV_1 is 50% of the total forced vital capacity (FVC)

D. Normal peak expiratory flow rate (PEFR) for men is about 450–700 l/min

E. A low vital capacity with normal PEFR and $\dfrac{FEV_1}{FVC}$ is typical of obstructive lung disease.

2.5. Which of the following are correct?

A. The function residual capacity is the same as the residual volume

B. The vital capacity is the sum of the expiratory reserve volume and the inspiratory reserve volume

C. Functional residual capacity can be measured by nitrogen washout

D. Residual volume is measured by spirometry

E. The normal residual volume is about 2 litres.

2.6. The compliance:

A. Is the reciprocal of the elastance

B. Is expressed in cmH_2O/l

C. Of the total chest is the sum of the compliances of the lungs and the thorax added together

D. Rises in the presence of pulmonary oedema

E. Rises during general anaesthesia.

Answers overleaf

2.4. A, D

The maximum volume of air that can be breathed in one minute is the maximum breathing capacity (MBC). Age and obstructive lung disease decrease MBC. MBC may be used to judge the effectiveness of bronchodilator therapy. FEV_1 signifies the forced expired volume in one second. It should be greater than 70% of the forced vital capacity. A FEV_1 of less than 70% indicates obstructive airways disease. The normal peak expiratory flow rate (PEFR) is less for adult women (300–500 l/min) than for men. A low value of PEFR indicates obstructive disease. A low vital capacity with normal PEFR and $\frac{FEV_1}{FVC}$ indicates restrictive lung disease.

2.5. C

The functional residual capacity is the volume of air in the lungs at the end of a normal expiration: the sum of the expiratory reserve volume and the residual volume. It can be determined by collecting and measuring all the nitrogen obtained during a period of oxygen breathing (nitrogen washout). It can also be determined using a whole body plethysmograph. The vital capacity is the sum of expiratory reserve volume and the inspiratory capacity (inspiratory capacity is tidal volume plus inspiratory reserve volume). Residual volume is calculated from functional residual capacity and expiratory reserve volume; it is normally about $1 \cdot 2$ l in males and $1 \cdot 1$ l in females.

2.6. A

Compliance, in l/cmH_2O, measures the elastic property of the lungs (as does the reciprocal, elastance, in cmH_2O/l). The lung alone (C_L), and the thorax alone (C_T), are naturally more compliant than both together (C_B). The compliance of the two is obtained by adding their elastances $\left(\frac{1}{C_B} = \frac{1}{C_L} + \frac{1}{C_T}\right)$. Pulmonary oedema and anaesthesia both reduce the compliance of the lung.

2.7. Surfactant:

A. Is made in type II alveolar cells
B. Is a lipoprotein
C. Is decreased in premature babies
D. Is decreased by increased FIo_2
E. Causes a decrease in surface tension as the alveoli expand.

2.8. When a lung is mechanically inflated and then allowed to deflate:

A. The pleural pressure gradient falls during inflation
B. Surfactant lowers the surface tension during deflation
C. Exhalation occurs principally due to recoil of the elastic fibres in the lung
D. Laplace's law is obeyed.
E. Hysteresis can be prevented by positive–end–expiratory–pressure.

2.9. Which of the following are true?

A. Normal intrapleural pressures range from -5.5 mmHg to -2.5 mmHg
B. With strong inspiratory effort against a closed glottis, pressures of -40 mmHg can be developed
C. Paradoxical respiration is seen with a flail chest
D. If the peak inspiratory pressure increases during mechanical ventilation a tension pneumothorax may exist
E. During spontaneous ventilation with an open pneumothorax the normal lung will fill with air from the contralateral lung as well as from the trachea.

Answers overleaf

2.7. A, B, C, D

As alveoli get smaller, surfactant causes a decrease in surface tension thus preventing complete collapse of the alveoli. Lack of adequate surfactant in the premature newborn is felt to be a major factor in development of the respiratory distress syndrome.

2.8. B

As the lung is stretched, its tendency to contract generates a larger gradient across the visceral pleura. The role of surfactant is to lower the surface tension, especially at low volumes. Nevertheless the surface tension forces are responsible for about 2/3 of the force encountered during inflation and provide most of the force during exhalation. If Laplace's law (pressure = 2 × surface tension/radius) were obeyed, surface tension effects would collapse the small airways and alveoli; surfactant prevents this. Hysteresis refers to the discrepancy between the pressure/volume relationship recorded during inspiration and that recorded during expiration; it is encountered when deforming many tissues and materials and is not prevented by PEEP.

2.9. All correct

Intrapleural pressure is always negative compared with intra-alveolar pressure; it is normally subatmospheric at rest, becomes markedly so during forced inspiration, but can rise to over 50 mmHg positive pressure during forced expiration. Paradoxical respiration means that the flail segment retracts when the rest of the chest expands, and expands during exhalation when the rest of the chest contracts. A tension pneumothorax compresses the lung necessitating an increase in inspiratory pressure to achieve the same tidal volume. During spontaneous ventilation with open pneumothorax the normal lung will draw air from the contralateral lung. During expiration the normal lung will empty into the contralateral lung. This phenomenon is sometimes called pendelluft or pendulum air. This amounts to rebreathing and causes an elevated P_{CO_2}.

2.10. Static compliance:

A. Is the change in volume per unit of pressure
B. Of the normal lung is 0.2 l/cm H_2O
C. Of the normal thoracic wall is 0.2 l/cm H_2O
D. Of lungs and thorax is 0.1 l/cm H_2O
E. Is measured when the breath is held.

2.11. In normal lung in the erect posture:

A. The blood flow is greatest in the base
B. The ventilation is greatest in the apex
C. The alveolar Po_2 is greatest at the apex
D. The alveolar Pco_2 is greatest at the apex
E. The capillary pH is closest to normal arterial values at the apex.

2.12. During normal quiet breathing:

A. The peripheral parts of the lung expand more than those near the hilum
B. The parts of the lungs near the diaphragm have greater ventilation than those at the apex
C. The external intercostal muscles raise the ribs
D. The abdominal muscles aid expiration
E. The scalene muscles are inactive.

2.13. West described zones in the lung on the basis of alveolar, arterial and venous pressure (PA, Pa, Pv):

A. Zone 1 is lung above the level where venous pressure equals alveolar pressure: $P\text{A} > P\text{v}$
B. Zone 2 is lung where the venous pressure lies between the arterial and alveolar pressures: $P\text{a} > P\text{v} > P\text{A}$
C. Zone 1 is normally about 1/9 of the lung volume
D. Positive end expiratory pressure (PEEP) tends to increase zone 1 and thus enlarge the dead space
E. Haemorrhagic shock decreases zone 1 thus decreasing the dead space.

Answers overleaf

2.10. All correct

If compliance is measured during breathing it is called dynamic compliance. Compliance will be changed by: interstitial oedema in congestive heart failure: loss of surfactant for any reason; changes in functional residual capacity; breakdown of elasticity of the lung; arthritic changes in the rib cage; retention of sputum; straining and many other factors.

2.11. A, C

Gravity directs most of the blood flow to the base. This heavy base, like a water-logged sponge, contains relatively less air than the apex. However, being least stretched, it yields most easily and receives most ventilation. The gradient of these relationships, from apex to base, affects blood flow more than ventilation; accordingly there is *relatively* more ventilation at the apex. The result is a higher PO_2 and pH and lower PCO_2 in the apical capillary.

2.12. A, B, C

Those parts of the lungs in contact with the mobile part of the thoracic cage (i.e. diaphragm and chest wall) expand the most. There is greater movement at the diaphragm than at the apex and therefore greater ventilation. The abdominal muscles play little, if any, part in normal quiet breathing. They do aid *forced* expiration. The scalene muscles contract with each inspiration, but produce a very small part of the tidal volume.

2.13. D

Zone 2 is lung where the alveolar pressure lies between the arterial and venous pressure ($Pa > PA > Pv$). Above this is zone 1 ($PA > Pa$) and below is zone 3 ($Pv > PA$). Zone 1 conditions are not present in normal people; if they are the apex is not perfused. PEEP enlarges zone 1 and thus enlarges the fraction of lung not perfused (i.e. dead space). Haemorrhagic shock has the same effect by reducing flow to the upper part of the lung.

2.14. Which of the following might appropriately be used in calculating the shunt fraction Qs/Qt?

    A. Haemoglobin
    B. Mixed venous P_{CO_2}
    C. Alveolar P_{O_2}
    D. Arterial P_{CO_2}
    E. Arterial pH.

2.15. In the normal resting 70 kg upright adult:

    A. Ventilation is greater at the apex than at the base
    B. Minute alveolar ventilation is 2 l and cardiac output is 3 l
    C. The normal ventilation/perfusion ratio is 1.5 for the whole lung
    D. The ventilation/perfusion ratio is 3.3 at the lung apex
    E. The ventilation/perfusion ratio is 0.63 at the lung base.

2.16. The oxygen dissociation curve of human haemoglobin has a characterisic S shape:

    A. Acidaemia shifts the curve to the left
    B. High P_{CO_2} shifts the curve to the right
    C. Hyperthermia shifts the curve to the left
    D. The curve for fetal haemoglobin is further to the right
    E. High levels of 2,3 DPG shift the curve to the left.

Answers overleaf

2.14. A, C

The ratio between the calculated shunt (Qs) and the cardiac output (Qt) = the ratio $\frac{(c-a)}{(c-v)}$ where c, a and v represent the capillary, arterial and mixed venous oxygen *contents*. The content is derived by multiplying the haemoglobin concentration by 1.39 and adding the amount of oxygen in solution (0.0031 × partial pressure). This equation assumes that the haemoglobin is fully saturated, i.e. 1 g carries 1.39 ml of oxygen.

2.15. D, E

Ventilation is greatest at the base of the lung. However the ventilation/perfusion ratio is high at the apex. Normal minute alveolar ventilation is 4 l, while cardiac output is about 5 l/min. The normal ventilation/perfusion ratio for the whole lung is 0.8 and is about 3.3 at the apex and 0.63 at the base.

2.16. B

It is helpful to remember that in active muscle there is heat, acidosis and an elevated $P\text{co}_2$; in this environment the curve moves right, i.e. a given level of saturation relates to a higher partial pressure. Oxygen is more readily available to the tissues. Fetal haemoglobin accepts more oxygen than adult haemoglobin at a given partial pressure, i.e. the fetal curve is to the left. Low levels of 2,3 DPG also shift the curve to the left (e.g. in banked blood). The Bohr effect is the shift to the right of the oxygen dissociation curve caused by acidosis. The Haldane effect describes the greater affinity of deoxygenated haemoglobin for carbon dioxide, the combined form being carbamino haemoglobin. Deoxygenated haemoglobin also takes up hydrogen ions formed by the dissociation of H_2CO_3.

2.17. Which of the following are true?

   A. Oxygen is an explosive gas

   B. The oxygen content of blood is the amount of oxygen that can be extracted from 100 ml of blood

   C. The oxygen capacity is calculated by dividing the oxygen content by the oxygen saturation

   D. Oxygen saturation $= \dfrac{O_2 \text{ content} - \text{dissolved } O_2}{O_2 \text{ capacity} - \text{dissolved } O_2} \times 100$

   E. The oxygen capacity is independent of the alveolar carbon dioxide partial pressure.

2.18. Which of the following are true?

   A. Methaemoglobinemia causes cyanosis, despite normal heart and lung function

   B. Methaemoglobinemia can be caused by drugs such as nitrites, nitrates, phenacetin and prilocaine

   C. Methaemoglobinemia can be treated by vitamin C or methylene blue (1–2 mg/kg)

   D. Carbon monoxide causes cyanosis by reducing the oxygen-carrying capacity of blood

   E. Cyanosis is not possible in anaemic patients whose blood contains less than 5 g/dl of haemoglobin.

2.19. Physiological responses to moderate hypoxia include:

   A. Tachycardia

   B. Decreased systemic vascular resistance

   C. Pulmonary vasoconstriction

   D. Increased circulating catecholamines

   E. Decreased Pa_{CO_2}.

Answers overleaf

2.17. B, D

Oxygen supports combustion, but cannot itself be ignited. The oxygen capacity is that volume of oxygen carried by 100 ml of blood saturated with room air. It includes both oxygen combined with haemoglobin and in physical solution.

Since the amount of oxygen combined with haemoglobin is effected by the P_{CO_2} (increased CO_2 shifts the curve to the right), the O_2 capacity will change with changes in P_{CO_2}.

2.18. A, B, C

Methaemoglobinemia and carbon monoxide exposure both reduce the oxygen carrying capacity of the blood. However, carboxyhaemoglobin is red, not blue. Methaemoglobinemia can be inherited or induced by drug exposure. Reducing agents can be effective therapy: vitamin C is effective in the treatment of the inherited form of methaemoglobinemia while methylene blue will treat both forms. Cyanosis will be evident when there is more than 5 g of deoxygenated haemoglobin per dl. Cyanosis can occur in severe anaemia, due either to injected dyes or to methaemoglobin, because only 1.5 g/dl of this pigment is needed to cause cyanosis.

2.19. All correct

The fall in P_{aCO_2} is secondary to hypoxic hyperventilation. The increased catecholamines cause tachycardia and a raised cardiac output. This, with the hypoxic pulmonary vasoconstriction, causes an increase in right ventricular pressure and work.

2.20. In normal man, breathing 100% O_2 at 3 atmospheres pressure (3 ATA):

A. 1 g of haemoglobin carries about 60 ml of O_2
B. The Pa_{O_2} would be about 2280 mmHg
C. The amount of O_2 in physical solution is 13.3 ml/100 ml blood
D. A mixed venous sample would have a haemoglobin saturation of 70%
E. A human could survive without any haemoglobin.

2.21. The CO_2 response curve:

A. Measures the cardiovascular response to CO_2
B. Is shifted to the left by morphine
C. Becomes steeper with hypoxia
D. Is shifted to the left by metabolic acidosis
E. Is shifted to the left by chronic obstructive lung disease.

Answers overleaf

2.20. E

Regardless of ambient pressure, 1 g of saturated haemoglobin carries 1.39 ml of oxygen per 100 ml of blood. However, raised pressure increases the amount of oxygen dissolved in plasma (0.003 ml O_2/100 ml blood/mmHg PaO_2). Breathing room air at sea level the PaO_2 would be about 100 mmHg, therefore 0.3 ml O_2 would be dissolved in 100 ml blood. At 3 atmospheres the PaO_2 approaches 2193 mmHg (2280-40-47) so the amount of dissolved oxygen approaches 6.6 ml per 100 ml of blood. Therefore, with any arteriovenous difference up to about 6 ml per 100 ml, there is adequate oxygen to sustain life without haemoglobin. This has been tested in animals and it was found that the venous blood remained oxygenated. In practice the presence of pulmonary shunt keeps the actual PaO_2 well below the theoretical maximum of 2193 mmHg. However, a human could, in theory, survive for a while without haemoglobin.

2.21. C, D

The CO_2 response curve plots minute ventilation (y–axis) against PCO_2 (x–axis). Either the slope of the curve may be altered, or it may be shifted to the right or left. A stimulus (i.e. hypoxia), which causes an increase in the slope, will increase the change in minute ventilation produced by a given PCO_2 change. A shift to the right (e.g. metabolic alkalosis) shows a decreased ventilatory response while a shift to the left (e.g. metabolic acidosis) shows an increased response.

Chronic obstructive lung disease causes a decrease in slope, thereby decreasing the minute ventilation at elevated PCO_2's. When the disease is severe enough to cause CO_2 retention the curve is also shifted to the right.

Narcotics and most inhalation agents depress ventilation. Morphine causes a shift to the right. Pethidine decreases the slope in addition to shifting the curve to the right. Halothane decreases the slope with increasing concentration until it almost becomes flat.

2.22. An elevation in Paco$_2$ results in:

A. An increased systolic BP
B. An increase in plasma catecholamines
C. An increase in surgical bleeding
D. An elevation in Pao$_2$
E. Increased blood flow to the brain.

2.23. Which of the following are true of carbon dioxide?

A. It is 20 times more diffusible than oxygen
B. Arterial blood normally carries 50 ml of carbon dioxide per 100 ml
C. Mixed venous Paco$_2$ is normally 46 mmHg
D. The reaction between CO_2 and H_2O is catalysed by carbonic anhydrase in the plasma
E. Arterial blood carries 6% of the carbon dioxide in the form of solution.

2.24. Which are true about respiratory tract reflexes?

A. The Hering–Breuer reflex makes the diaphram stop contracting when the lungs are inflated
B. The deflation reflex cause an increased rate and force of inspiration
C. The reflex of Head causes a strong diaphragmatic contraction when lungs are inflated during partial vagus blockade
D. Aspiration of secretions causes reflex glottic closure and bronchoconstriction
E. Stimulation of the J-receptor cause tachypnoea.

Answers overleaf

2.22. A, B, C, E

Elevated Pa_{CO_2} causes release of catecholamines, thereby elevating blood pressure and cardiac output; surgical bleeding is often increased due to capillary dilation. Cerebral vessels dilate in response to increased Pa_{CO_2} and constrict in response to decreased Pa_{CO_2}. In the presence of increased intracranial pressure, respiratory depressants should not be given unless ventilation is adequately maintained; hyperventilation reduces incracranial pressure. Elevation of Pa_{CO_2} tends to lower Pa_{O_2}; the two gases compete for space in the alevoli and an elevation of one takes place at the expense of the other.

2.23. A, B, C, E

Carbonic anhydrase is the catalyst for the reaction:

$$CO_2 + H_2O \rightleftharpoons H_2CO_3$$

However this reaction takes place in the red blood cell, not the plasma. In arterial blood most of the carbon dioxide is carried as bicarbonate and in combination with haemoglobin; only 6% is in physical solution.

2.24. All correct

The Hering–Breuer or inflation reflex results from stimulation of stretch receptors. It is doubtful if this reflex exists in man. Receptors in the alveoli and bronchioles sense deflation and cause an inspiratory effort to be made. The reflex of Head does not occur when the vagus nerve is intact or when it is completely blocked. Receptors that sense irritation, such as aspiration, are located in the larynx at the carina and other sites where the bronchi branch. The J-receptors or juxta-pulmonary capillary receptors are found in the alveolar walls. They react to pulmonary oedema and emboli with resultant tachypnoea.

2.25. Assuming normal atrioventricular conduction the heart rate is determined by:

  A. Serum renin levels
  B. The rhythmicity of the sinoatrial node
  C. The parasympathetic nervous system
  D. The sympathetic nervous system
  E. The myocardial fibres' preload.

2.26. In the electrocardiogram (ECG):

  A. Standard lead I is right arm to left leg
  B. The PR interval is normally no longer than 0.12 seconds
  C. The QRS should normally be less than 0.10 seconds
  D. High-peaked T waves are characteristic of elevated serum potassium levels
  E. U waves are associated with low calcium levels.

2.27. Which are true concerning ventricular preload?

  A. The end-diastolic pressure is related to fibre length
  B. The ventricular stroke output is inversely related to the initial fibre length
  C. Preload is influenced by myocardial contractility
  D. Preload is influenced by ventricular afterload
  E. The diastolic atrial pressure is the only direct measurement of preload.

Answers overleaf

2.25. B, C, D

The heart rate is primarily determined by the spontaneously depolarizing cells in the sinoatrial (SA) node. If the SA node fails, the atrioventrical node or ventricular cells will pace as they also spontaneously depolarize. The SA node dominates because it has the fastest rate of depolarization.

The autonomic nervous system can modify the heart rate. Parasympathetic stimulation (via the vagus) cause slowing, while sympathetic stimulation (via the cardiac accelerator fibres of T1 to T4) increase the heart rate.

2.26. C, D

The normal 12-lead ECG has three standard bipolar leads (I,II,III) three augmented unipolar lead (AVR, AVL, AVF) and six unipolar chest leads. The normal range for the PR interval is 0.12–0.20 seconds. If the QRS is longer than 0.10 seconds, intraventricular conduction defects should be expected.

High-peaked T waves are characteristic of elevated potassium levels. They are also seen in posterior myocardial infarction, acute anterior myocardial infarction, severe aortic stenosis, and left ventricular hypertrophy.

The U wave is thought to be the repolarization of the T wave. It is usually not noticeable. However with hypokalaemia it becomes prominent.

2.27. A, C, D

Preload is the tension of the myocardial fibre in end-diastole. The only *direct* indicator of preload is the fibre length. Measurement of left atrial pressure, pulmonary capillary wedge pressure, right atrial pressure, or central venous pressure, are used clinically to approximate the preload.

Factors which affect preload are the vascular blood volume, the venous tone, the contractile state of the heart and ventricular after load.

2.28. The afterload of the heart:

    A. Changes with changing preload
    B. Is the tension the myocardium is called upon to develop during contraction
    C. Is inversely proportional to the arterial blood pressure for a given preload and myocardial contractility.
    D. Directly influences the stroke volume
    E. Is greater in heart failure.

2.29. Which of the following pressures (in mmHg) are normal:

    A. Right atrium—15
    B. Right ventricle—20/4
    C. Left atrium—20
    D. Left ventricular end-diastolic—16
    E. Pulmonary artery wedge pressure—20.

2.30. Stroke volume

    A. Is one determinant of cardiac output
    B. Is affected by preload
    C. Is independent of myocardial contractility
    D. Is related to afterload
    E. Is principally determined by the heart rate.

Answers overleaf

2.28. A, B, E

In the intact heart, afterload is determined by cavity pressure (which changes with preload) and the ventricular radius. Since a failing heart has a greater radius, the afterload is higher in heart failure. A rise in blood pressure increases afterload, which decreases stroke volume, thus tending to maintain a steady blood pressure.

2.29. B

The range of normal pressure is:

Location	mmHg
Right atrium	0–10
Right ventricle	$\frac{15–30}{0–8}$
Pulmonary artery	$\frac{15–30}{5–15}$
Pulmonary artery wedge	5–15
Left atrium	4–12
Left ventricle	$\frac{100–120}{5–15}$
Left ventricle end-diastolic	4–12

2.30. A, B, D

The cardiac output (CO) is equal to the stroke volume (SV) times the heart rate (HR): CO = SV × HR. The stroke volume is directly related to the preload and myocardial contractility and inversely to the afterload. In fact, it is now common practice to reduce afterload by vasodilation to achieve an increased stroke volume and therefore improve cardiac output.

2.31. Myocardial oxygen consumption is:

A. Normally about 25 ml/min
B. Increased by raising the FIo_2
C. Increased by greater left ventricular wall tension
D. Decreased by a raised peripheral venous pressure
E. Inversely proportional to the heart rate.

2.32. Venous return to the heart:

A. Is not influenced by arterial pressure
B. Is increased by the pumping action of muscles
C. Is decreased during spontaneous inspiration
D. Is increased by the suction-like action of the ventricular muscles
E. Is increased by the pumping action of the venous system.

2.33. The mean arterial blood pressure (MAP):

A. Is important because it determines the mean blood flow to an organ
B. Is calculated at normal heart rate by the formula:

$$MAP = \frac{\text{Systolic blood pressure} + \text{diastole blood pressure}}{2}$$

C. Can be measured by attaching an indwelling arterial catheter to a mercury manometer
D. Can be obtained by measuring or calculating the area under a pressure curve
E. Maintains a constant relationship with the mean venous pressure (MVP) such that MAP–MVP = 62.

Answers overleaf

2.31. A, C

The heart normally extracts 10–12 ml of oxygen from every 100 ml of blood and coronary blood flow is 250 ml/min. This extraction rate is high compared to other metabolically active organs, such as the liver (2.5–4.5 ml) or the kidney (2–4 ml).

Increased myocardial contractility, heart rate or the left ventricular wall tension all raise the myocardial oxygen consumption.

2.32. B, D

Factors influencing venous return are (1) arterial pressure, (2) gravity, (3) muscle pumping action, (4) the abdominal–thoracic pump, (5) the heart action, (6) venomotor tone and (7) the integrity of the venous valves.

Arterial pressure provides a force from behind after the blood has passed through the capillaries. Pressure in the capillaries is about 15 mmHg; this falls to about 10 mmHg in the peripheral veins. While the head down position does not augment venous return and cardiac output, gravity can help if the trunk is kept level and the legs raised. Muscle pumping action is important in returning blood against a gradient. During inspiration the intrathoracic pressure falls and abdominal pressure increases to cause blood to flow from the abdomen to the chest and is called the abdominal–thoracic pump. The ventricular muscle exerts a suction-like effect on the venous system. Finally, while the veins have no pumping action themselves, venoconstriction provides a favourable gradient for venous return.

2.33. A, C, D

At normal heart rates:

MAP = Diastolic BP + 1/3 (systolic BP – diastolic BP)

At very rapid heart rates the MAP will approach 1/2 the pulse pressure:

$$\text{MAP} = \frac{\text{Systolic BP} + \text{Diastolic BP}}{2}$$

MAP has no constant relationship to MVP.

2.34. Capillaries

A. Increase their blood flow in response to local hypoxia
B. Exchange solutes with the tissues as a result of concentration gradients
C. Exchange solutes with the tissues as a result of capillary permeability
D. Tend to gain fluid because of plasma osmotic pressure
E. Tend to gain fluid because of hydrostatic pressure.

2.35. In the peripheral circulation:

A. The capacitance vessels are the primary determinants of vascular resistance
B. Vascular beds are considered to be in parallel
C. The total peripheral resistance is always less than any individual bed
D. Resistance is most dramatically affected by the length of a vessel
E. The beds with the highest resistance have the greatest effect on the total resistance.

2.36. Which of the following are true?

A. The vessel rich group of organs receives about 70% of the cardiac output
B. The muscle group receives 50% of the cardiac output
C. The fat receives 25% of the cardiac output
D. The vessel poor group of organs receives 10% of the cardiac output.

Answers overleaf

2.34. A, B, C

The precapillary sphincter dilates with local hypoxia, resulting in more oxygen delivery to the hypoxic site. Solutes, such as hydrogen ions, electrolytes and even proteins in small amounts, are exchanged with the tissues as a result of capillary permeability and concentration gradients. Osmotic pressure is largely irrelevant to the capillary wall as small molecules pass freely across the membrane. The larger molecules are responsible for the oncotic pressure (colloid osmotic pressure). Hydrostatic pressure tends to force fluid out of the capillaries aided by tissue oncotic pressure. Plasma oncotic pressure tends to hold fluid in the capillaries aided by tissue hydrostatic pressure. The balance of these forces ultimately determines where fluid is gained and lost in the capillary bed.

2.35. B, C

In the peripheral circulation the most important determinants of vascular resistance are the small arterioles (10–15 μ diameter) in which the greatest pressure drop occurs. The capacitance vessels, the veins, contain 65–75% of the total blood volume. Since all beds are considered to be in parallel, the bed with the *lowest* resistance has the greatest effect on total resistance.

The resistance through any given vessel is most affected by its radius according to Poiseuille's equation:

$$\text{Resistance} = \frac{8LV}{\pi r^4}$$

(where L = length, V = viscosity, r = radius)

2.36. A

The brain, heart, liver and kidneys receive about 70% of the cardiac output. They are the first organs significantly affected by anaesthetic drugs. The drugs are redistributed to the muscle and skin, which receive about 25% of the cardiac output, and to the fat which receives 6% of the cardiac output. The vessel poor group, consisting of bone, ligaments and cartilage, receive very little blood flow.

2.37. Autoregulation of blood flow:

    A. Provides a constant blood flow at different pressures
    B. May result from fluid leaking into the tissues, which puts pressure on the vessel and slows the flow through it
    C. May result from smooth muscle contraction in response to increased intraluminal pressure
    D. Is not related to tissue metabolism
    E. Is responsive to sympathetic stimulation.

2.38. Coronary artery blood flow:

    A. Occurs predominantly during systole
    B. Is less adequate in the presence of tachycardia
    C. Is predominantly controlled by α and β stimulation of the sympathetic nervous system
    D. Is about 50 ml/min in the normal adult
    E. Is not normally influenced by changes in cardiac tissue metabolism.

Answers overleaf

2.37. A, B, C

The *Tissue Pressure Theory* of autoregulation indicates that tissue pressure compresses the vessel and thus decreases flow through it. The *Myogenic Hypothesis* states that vascular smooth muscle contracts in response to pressure in the vessel. This decreases flow by the fourth power of the radius. The *Metabolic Theory* states that a decrease in flow causes a decreased oxygen tension in the vessel which causes vasodilation. Although the actual substances have not been identified, possibilities are: hydrogen ions, potassium ions, adenosine, lactic acid, histamine or acetylcholine.

2.38. B

70–90% of coronary artery flow occurs during diastole when there is low intramural resistance. Since tachycardia shortens diastole, and also increases myocardial oxygen consumption, it decreases the adequacy of the coronary blood flow.

The normal flow is about 250 ml/min and is controlled mainly by local metabolic factors, especially tissue hypoxia and acidosis. There is sympathetic innervation, but it plays a minor role in controlling the blood flow.

Physiology

2.39. Which of the following are true about blood pressure regulating receptors and reflexes?

A. Baroreceptors and chemoreceptors play an important role in chronic regulation of blood pressure
B. High pressure baroreceptor stimulation causes vasodilation
C. Low pressure baroreceptors are activated at systolic blood pressures below 1 mmHg
D. Chemoreceptors located in the carotid and aortic body have little effect on blood pressure
E. Chemoreceptors in the vasomotor centre are the most powerful known stimulators of the sympathetic nervous system.

2.40. The electroencephalogram (EEG)

A. Records brain wave potentials in the 3–5 volt range
B. May contain alpha, theta and delta waves in normal individuals
C. Is generally 'flat' during siezure activity
D. Will show rapid low amplitude activity during hypoxia
E. At brain temperatures of 20°C shows little activity in the parietal or occipital regions.

Answers overleaf

2.39. B, E

Baroreceptors and chemoreceptors are important in the acute control of blood pressure, but tend to adapt with time. Chronic control occurs through changes in blood volume.

High pressure baroreceptors in the carotid and aortic sinuses send impulses to the pons and medulla. The result of stimulation is a slowing of the heart rate and decrease in the stength of cardiac contraction and peripheral vasodilatation.

Low pressure baroreceptors in the right and left atria, pulmonary artery and perhaps the great veins and ventricular walls are stimulated by overfilling. Afferent impulses to the medulla produce peripheral vasodilatation and thereby decrease venous return to the heart.

Chemoreceptors are primarily involved with control of respiration; however they also affect circulation when the blood pressure is low. The chemoreceptors in the carotid and aortic bodies respond when pressures fall below 80 mmHg. Those in the vasomotor centre start functioning at pressures below 65 mmHg. If the pressures fall to 20–30 mmHg they provide the most powerful sympathetic stimulation known, increasing cardiac contractility and causing maximal arteriolar and venous constriction. The action of the chemoreceptors is most likely stimulated by the ischaemia that results from low blood flow.

2.40. B, E

The normal EEG records brain potentials of about 10 microvolts. Normal waves are: delta 0.5–3.5 Hz, 100 microvolts amplitude; theta 4–7 Hz, 50 microvolts amplitude, and alpha 8–13 Hz, 75 microvolts amplitude.

During seizure activity 'spikes' of moderate amplitude group together followed by slow waves of 1.5–3 Hz.

Hypoxia causes slow waves (1–3 Hz) of increased amplitude. The effect of hypothermia depends on the temperature. At 32°C a slight decrease in amplitude and frequency occurs; at 25°C a lower amplitude is seen, at 20°C little activity is seen in the parietal and occipital areas while low amplitude slow waves are recorded in the frontal area.

2.41. A raised intracranial pressure (ICP) can be lowered by increasing:

    A. Cerebral blood flow
    B. The rate of CSF production
    C. The inspired CO_2 tension
    D. The rate of CSF absorption
    E. Central venous pressure.

2.42. Cerebrospinal fluid (CSF):

    A. Is formed in the arachnoid villi
    B. Is absorbed in the choroid plexus
    C. Has a total volume of 120 ml in the average adult
    D. Contains about 60 mg/dl of glucose
    E. Has a sodium content of 40 mmol/l.

2.43. Which of the following are true of the neuromuscular junction?

    A. It includes both the pre- and post-synaptic area
    B. The junctional folds contain a high concentration of cholinesterase
    C. The junctional folds contain the sodium pores
    D. Acetylcholine receptor sites are around the sodium pores
    E. Acetylcholine is inactivated by passing through the sodium pores.

2.44. In the resting state, at the motor end plate:

    A. There is normally zero millivolts potential
    B. The intracellular to extracellular potassium ratio is about 40 to 1
    C. The sodium pump maintains a high intracellular sodium concentration
    D. Sodium has one-fiftieth (1/50) the permeability of potassium
    E. The transmembrane potential is predominantly dependent on potassium.

Answers overleaf

2.41. D

Of the total intracranial volume, 10% is cerebrospinal fluid (CSF) and 4% is blood. A raised ICP reduces cerebral blood flow and alters the CSF dynamics; both the CSF rate of absorption is increased and its production decreased. An elevated Pa_{CO_2} and central venous pressure both increase ICP. Normal ICP is 10–15 mmHg. There can be a considerable increase in the volume of the intracranial contents before the ICP starts to rise because of the displacement of blood and CSF referred to above.

2.42. C, D

CSF is formed in the cerebral ventricles, probably by the choroid plexus. It is reabsorbed by the arachnoid villi. Rate of formation is about 350–700 ml/min and the total volume is about 100–150 ml. CSF contains: 138 mmol/l sodium, 2.8 mmol/l potassium, 124 mmol/l chloride, 60 mg/dl glucose and 25 mg/dl protein.

2.43. A, B, C, D

The junctional folds occur as infoldings along the course of the nerve ending on the myofibril. The sodium pores are in this area and there is, here, a high concentration of cholinesterase. The sodium pores are thought to contain acetylcholine receptor sites. The attachment of acetylcholine deforms the pores and allows sodium to pass in and depolarization to take place. The acetylcholine is rapidly destroyed by the cholinesterase in the area.

2.44. B, D, E

The transmembrane potential depends mainly on the most permeable ion; at rest, it is potassium. However, when electrical activity is initiated, sodium permeability increases. The sodium pump removes sodium from the cell against a gradient. The normal resting potential is about -90 millivolts.

2.45. Acetylcholine

A. Is formed by the acetylation of choline in the presence of cholinesterase
B. Is stored in packets in the nerve endings
C. Causes an action potential to occur as the result of multiple miniature end-plate potentials
D. Is liberated in reduced amounts in the presence of increased magnesium concentration
E. Is liberated in reduced amounts in the presence of aminoglycoside antibiotics.

2.46. In normal muscle contraction:

A. Calcium ions are released when the myofibril depolarizes
B. Heat and energy are produced in the muscle by release of phosphate from ATP
C. ATP causes relaxation of muscle fibres
D. Calcium ions are stored in the sarcoplasmic reticulum
E. Excess calcium uncouples oxidative phosphorylation.

2.47. A sarcomere contains:

A. A lines
B. B bands
C. C bands
D. Z lines
E. F lines

Answers overleaf

2.45. B, D, E

Acetylcholine is the transmitter at the neuromuscular junction. It is formed by the acetylation of choline in the presence of *choline acetylase*. It is then contained in quanta or packets in the nerve ending. Small amounts of acetylcholine are released continuously and this results in miniature end-plate potentials which can be measured but are too small to cause muscle contraction. Aminoglycosides, decreased calcium and increased magnesium all decrease the amount of acetylcholine released.

2.46. All correct

Calcium ions are stored in the sarcoplasmic reticulum and released on depolarization. They are normally reaccumulated in the sarcoplasmic reticulum by means of a calcium pump. The release of calcium ions causes the activation of ATP–ase, which in turn initiates the loss of phosphate from ATP to provide energy for the contraction. ATP is reformed in the mitochondria. The increased level of ATP causes relaxation of the muscle fibre.

2.47. D

A sarcomere is a unit of myofibril. It contains A and I bands. The I bands contain actin, the A bands contain myosin and the enzyme ATPase. The actin and myosin bands interdigitate to shorten the fibre length. The Z line is part of an aqueous channel system that carries the excitation impulse from the motor end plate to the inside of the muscle. The system passes close to the sarcoplasmic reticulum. When carrying excitation impulses, it causes the sarcoplasmic reticulum to liberate Ca^{++} which in turn triggers ATPase to act on ATP to release energy for muscle contraction.

2.48. The 'gate control theory of pain' states that:

A. Painful stimuli inhibit the transmitter neurons or target cells (T-cells)
B. Large nerve fibres inhibit the substantia gelatinosa cells (SG cells)
C. Small nerve fibres activate the SG cells
D. The SG cell inhibits the T cell
E. Cerebral control is lacking in pain perception.

2.49. Pain sensation

A. Is carried in C nerve fibres
B. Is carried in A-delta nerve fibres
C. From skin, muscle and bones goes to the dorsal horn of the spinal cord
D. From skin, muscle and bones leaves the dorsal horn cell and travels up to the cord in the ipsilateral spinothalamic tract
E. From skin, muscle and tissues may go through the reticular formation to the thalamus.

2.50. In the autonomic nervous system:

A. Noradrenaline is the sympathetic preganglionic neurotransmitter
B. Acetylcholine is the postganglionic sympathetic neurotransmitter for sweat glands
C. Acetylcholine is the postganglionic parasympathetic neurotransmitter
D. Noradrenaline is primarily inactivated by catechol-o-methyltransferase (COMT)
E. Adrenaline is the neurotransmitter in the α fibres of the sympathetic system

Answers overleaf

Physiology

2.48. D

In the 'gate control theory' both large and small fibres from the periphery act on the T cells and the SG cells. Activation of the SG cell inhibits the T cell and thus closes the gate for pain travelling up the cord. The small fibres inhibit the SG cell, thus allowing transmission of pain. However, while the large fibres carry impulses to the T cells they also stimulate the substantia gelatinosa which tends to close 'the gate'. Central control can also open and close the gate, thus modifying painful stimuli.

2.49. A, B, C, E

Pain is carried by A-delta fibres, the smallest of the myelinated somatic fibres, and by unmyelimated C fibres to the dorsal horn of the spinal cord. From there it is transmitted via the lateral spinothalamic tract of the *opposite* side of the cord. From the lateral spinothalamic tract the pain sensation travels either directly, or via the reticular formation, to the thalamus. Finally, the sensation is carried to the cortex via thalamocortical projections.

2.50. B, C

The preganglionic neurotransmitter for both the sympathetic and parasympathetic system is acetylcholine. It is also the postganglionic parasympathetic transmitter and the sympathetic postganglionic transmitter for sweat glands and vessels in skeletal muscles. Noradrenaline is the neurotransmitter at all other sympathetic postganglionic sites. Acetylcholine's action is terminated by acetylcholinesterase. Noradrenaline's action is terminated primarily by re-uptake into the nerve ending. COMT and monamine oxidase (MAO) metabolize what is not taken up.

2.51. In the autonomic nervous system:

A. Stimulation of the β-parasympathetic receptors in the heart causes tachycardia
B. Stimulation of the parasympathetic receptors in the gut increases intestinal motility
C. Stimulation of the α-sympathetic receptors in the blood vessels causes vasodilation
D. Stimulation of β_2-receptors causes bronchoconstriction
E. Pain can be carried by parasympathetic, but not sympathetic afferents.

2.52. Normal liver metabolism includes:

A. Formation and storage of glycogen
B. The breakdown of fats into glycerol and fatty acids
C. The production of renin
D. The production of prothrombin
E. The production of angiotensin.

2.53. Glomerular filtration:

A. Averages about 25 ml/min
B. Is about 20% of the total flow through the glomeruli
C. Produces a filtrate that is like plasma without the proteins
D. Results from the 'filtration pressure' which is equal to the mean arterial pressure
E. Occurs through a membrane which is less porous than the normal muscle capillary.

2.54. In the renal tubule:

A. 50% of the filtrate is returned to the circulation
B. Sodium is actively transported to the peritubular fluid
C. Water is reabsorbed by active transport
D. Sodium and chloride reabsorption takes place rapidly in the ascending loop of Henle
E. The permeability of the distal part is controlled by antidiuretic hormone (ADH).

Answers overleaf

2.51. B

The autonomic nervous system contains α- and β-sympathetic and parasympathetic divisions. The parasympathetics *are not* divided into α and β receptors. Parasympathetic stimulation causes bradycardia, constriction of the gut, constriction of the pupil of the eye, constriction of the bladder and penile erection. Alpha sympathetic stimulation causes vasoconstriction. β_1 stimulation increases the force and rate of cardiac contraction while β_2 stimulation causes vasodilation and bronchodilation.

2.52. A, B, D

The liver converts glucose to glycogen. The glycogen is stored and can then be used for energy (glycogenolysis). Fats are also broken down in the liver. Amino acids are synthesized to protein in the liver or converted to ammonia. Fats and proteins are also stored in the liver. The liver also produces prothrombin, fibrinogen and heparin. Renin is secreted by the juxtaglomerular cells in the kidney and converts angiotensinogen into angiotensin I. This is converted into the active vasopressor angiotensin II mainly by lung enzymes.

2.53. B, C

Filtration occurs through the glomerular membrane, which is much more porous than the average capillary and a much greater fraction of the plasma leaves the vessel. The average rate is 125 ml/min and this represents 20% of the total flow through the glomeruli and is called 'filtration fraction'. All of the blood, except cellular components and protein, are filtered. The filtration pressure is equal to the glomerular capillary pressure minus the sum of the glomerular colloid osmotic pressure and the pressure in Bowman's capsule.

2.54. B, D, E

Almost 99% of the filtrate is reabsorbed from the renal tubule. Sodium is actively transported while water follows passively. Sodium and chloride reabsorption is rapid in the ascending loop of Henle, which is almost impermeable to water. The permeability of the distal tubule increases in the presence of ADH.

2.55. The pituitary gland secretes:

- **A.** Antidiuretic hormone
- **B.** Oestrogens
- **C.** Androgens
- **D.** Growth hormone
- **E.** Insulin.

2.56. The thyroid gland:

- **A.** Normally produces thyroxine (T_4) and triidothyronine (T_3)
- **B.** Needs iodine from the diet to produce hormones
- **C.** Releases hormones in response to thyrotrophin (TSH)
- **D.** Is not influenced by activity of the hypothalamus
- **E.** Normally relies on long-acting thyroid stimulating hormone (LATS) to initiate hormone release

2.57. Physiologic effects of excess thyroxine levels include:

- **A.** Depression of the basal metabolic rate in the elderly
- **B.** Increased gut motility
- **C.** A feeling of tiredness (if excessive)
- **D.** Increased heart rate
- **E.** Generalized vasolidation.

Answers overleaf

2.55. A, D

The pituitary gland (also known as the hypophysis) is physiologically divided into two parts. The anterior pituitary gland (adenohypophysis) secretes growth hormone, corticotrophin, thyrotrophin, follicle-stimulating hormone, luteinizing hormone, luteotrophic hormone and melanocyte-stimulating hormone. The posterior pituitary (neurohypophysis) secretes antidiuretic hormone and oxytocin.

2.56. A, B, C

In addition to T_3 and T_4 the thyroid also secretes thyrocalcitonin in response to elevated calcium concentration in the blood. The thyroid gland depends on dietary iodine to produce T_3 and T_4. These hormones are released in response to thyrotrophin (TSH) from the anterior pituitary. TSH is released in response to thyroid-releasing hormone (TRH) from the hypothalamus. LATS is an abnormal TSH-like hormone that can be found in about 80% of patients with thyrotoxicosis.

2.57. B, C, D, E

The normal effects of thyroid hormones are generally stimulatory. Basal metabolic rate, heart rate, cardiac output, rate and depth of respiration, rate of secretion and motility of the gastrointestinal tract, and the activity of the central nervous system are all increased. Because of the increased metabolism there is generalized vasodilation. Tiredness develops in response to elevated levels of thyroxine because excess central nervous system stimulation impairs sleep. In the hyperthyroid state all of the above functions are exaggerated.

2.58. The adrenal gland secretes:

    A. Adrenaline and noradrenaline from its cortex
    B. Progesterone from its medulla
    C. Oestrogens from its cortex
    D. Androgens from its medulla
    E. Glucocorticoids from its cortex.

2.59. Which is true of adrenocorticosteroids?

    A. Mineralocorticoids increase renal sodium loss
    B. Mineralocorticoids increase renal potassium loss
    C. Glucocorticoids stimulate gluconeogenesis by the liver
    D. Glucocorticoids stimulate protein anabolism
    E. Glucocorticoids increase storage of adipose tissue.

2.60. The adrenal cortex is stimulated to increase secretion by:

    A. Corticosterone
    B. Intense heat
    C. Sympathomimetic drugs
    D. Trauma
    E. Intense cold.

Answers overleaf

2.58. C, E

The adrenal gland has two distinct parts, the adrenal medulla and the adrenal cortex. The *adrenal medulla* is functionally part of the sympathetic nervous system and secretes adrenaline and noradrenaline in response to sympathetic stimulation. The *adrenal cortex* secretes corticosteroids—the mineralocorticoids and the glucocorticoids. Androgens, oestrogens and progesterone are also produced in very small amounts in normal conditions. In pathologic states production of these sex hormones may be greatly increased resulting in either masculinization or feminization.

2.59. B, C, E

Mineralocorticoids influence the electrolytes of the extracellular fluids. They increase renal reabsorption of sodium and increase renal excretion of potassium. Cortisol comprises 95% of the glucocorticoids produced; its activity mainly controls metabolism. Gluconeogenesis is stimulated. Amino acids are mobilized from the tissues by protein catabolism and their utilization in the liver is enhanced. Even though cortisol increase the mobilization of fatty acids from adipose tissue, the rate of formation of fatty acids from glucose and amino acids by the adipose tissue is increased. At times the gain can be greater than the loss and therefore the amount of adipose tissue increases.

2.60. B, C, D, E

The adrenal cortex secretion is stimulated by adrenocorticotrophic hormone (ACTH) from the adenohypophysis. Corticosterone is one of the glucocorticoids secreted by the adrenal cortex. Stresses causing increased ACTH release, and thus increased adrenocortical secretion, include trauma, intense heat or cold, sympathomimetic drugs, debilitating disease, and restraining an animal so that it cannot move.

Physiology

2.61. During pregnancy:

A. The blood volume rises continuously until delivery
B. The central venous pressure rises progressively till term
C. The cardiac output reaches a maximum at 30–34 weeks
D. The systemic vascular resistance increases progressively till term
E. The venous capacity decreases progressively to term.

2.62. The supine pregnant patient in her last trimester:

A. Will increase her venous return to her heart
B. May increase her systemic vascular resistance
C. Will most likely reduce blood flow to the uterus
D. Will increase cardiac output
E. Will have aortocaval compression.

2.63. During labour:

A. Myocardial oxygen consumption increases
B. Hyperventilation shifts the oxygen dissociation curve to the left
C. There is an increase in circulating catecholamines
D. Blood pressure may fall during bearing down
E. Heart rate slows.

Answers overleaf

Physiology

2.61. C

The red cell and plasma volume, and therefore the total blood volume, increase until 30–34 weeks when a maximum is reached. This increased blood volume is contained in dilated veins of the uterus, kidneys, skeletal muscle and skin. The central venous pressure remains normal. The cardiac output increases to a maximum at 30–34 weeks; the blood pressure remains the same because the systemic vascular resistance falls.

2.62. B, C, E

Compression of the aorta and vena cava usually occur in the last trimester in the supine position. Caval compression decreases the venous return to the heart with a resultant fall in blood pressure, presumably due to decreased cardiac output. This is partially compensated for by a rise in systemic vascular resistance. Aortic compression reduces blood flow to the uterus and placenta. If the patient must lie on her back, as for a Caesarean section, the uterus should be manually displaced to the left to relieve the aortocaval compression.

2.63. A, B, C, D

During labour a great workload is placed on the cardiovascular system. Cardiac output, blood pressure and heart rate increase. However, with prolonged bearing down, the blood pressure may fall. The oxygen dissociation curve is shifted to the left by low P_{aCO_2}. Catecholamine levels are elevated and this may decrease the blood flow to the uterus. Even though labour and delivery seem to be something of a physiological trespass, the outcome is remarkably successful.

2.64. Which of the following are true?

   A. The fetus at term has a blood volume of 80 ml/kg

   B. The neonatal blood volume, 72 hours after birth, ranges from 75–107 ml/kg

   C. The neonate takes 3 days to establish its functional residual capacity

   D. Compression of the fetal chest, as it passes through the vagina, tends to collapse the lungs, adversely affecting the onset of spontaneous respiration

   E. A newborn develops a maximum negative pressure of -20 cmH$_2$O when initiating spontaneous respiration.

2.65. Normal arterial blood gas values during labour are:

   A. Fetal scalp vein pH = 7.32

   B. Umbilical vein PO_2 = 25 mmHg (3.3 kPa)

   C. Umbilical vein P_{CO_2} = 40 mmHg (5.3 kPa)

   D. Umbilical artery PO_2 = 70 mmHg (9.3 kPa)

   E. Umbilical artery P_{CO_2} = 50 mmHg (6.7 kPa).

Answers overleaf

2.64. A, B

The neonate's blood volume after birth varies between 75 and 107 ml/kg, depending on the amount of transfusion received from the placenta. Prolonging the interval from birth to clamping the umbilical cord, and lowering the neonate below the level of the placenta, both raise the neonate's blood volume. Chest compression during passage through the vagina helps squeeze fluid out of the lungs, and rebound from this compression draws air into the lungs. Both these effects are beneficial in initiating spontaneous respiration. Other factors that help to initiate respiration are acidosis, hypoxia, hypercarbia, cold, tactile stimulation and umbilical cord clamping.

The neonate has to develop a negative (or sub-atmospheric) pressure of -40 to -80 cmH$_2$O to overcome the elastic forces of the lungs and the surface tension of the collapsed alveoli. The functional residual capacity is established in the first hour after birth.

2.65. A, B, C, E

The correct values for fetal blood gases are:

	pH	Pa_{CO_2}	PO_2	O$_2$SAT%
Umbilical vein	7.30–7.35	38–42 mmHg (5.3 kPa)	26–32 mmHg (4 kPa)	70
Umbilical artery	7.24–7.29	48–54 mmHg (6.7 kPa)	12–18 mmHg (2 kPa)	28

The umbilical artery PO_2 represents the tension which was driving oxygen into the tissues. The average tissue PO_2 is therefore less than this, e.g. 10 mmHg, and in the mitochondria is considerably less still.

Sampling the pH of fetal scalp blood is one way of monitoring fetal wellbeing. The pH should normally be between 7.25–7.35. A pH below 7.25 gives cause for concern; below 7.20 is an indication for urgent delivery, especially with other signs of fetal distress (e.g. bradycardia).

Physiology

2.66. During surface cooling to produce hypothermia:

  A. The hypothalamic temperature-regulating centre responds
     to a fall in blood temperature as small as 0.2°C
  B. The metabolic rate is halved at 30°C
  C. The rectal temperature is the closest representation of core
     temperature
  D. Carbon dioxide becomes less soluble in the blood
  E. The blood pressure is elevated between 35°C and 29°C due
     to peripheral vasoconstriction.

Answers overleaf

2.66. None correct

The hypothalamic centre responds to changes of 0.5°C. At 30°C the metabolic rate has fallen to about 0.75 normal. The 'core' temperature is not well represented by any central temperature. Long after cooling is withdrawn, the cold skin and fat will be equilibrating and cooling the rest of the body. The oesophageal temperature reflects such changes better, being close to blood returning to the heart; the rectal temperature will be slower to respond. All gases are more soluble in colder solvents. Blood pressure falls slightly during hypothermia.

3. PHYSICS

3.1. A normal value for atmospheric pressure at sea level would be:

A. 760 mmHg
B. 10 332 mm H_2O
C. 14.69 lb in^{-2} (p.s.i.)
D. 101 325 N m^{-2}
E. 101.3 kPa.

3.2. The pressure changes as gas passes from a full cylinder of gas through various valves and enters the breathing circuit. The following pressures are typical in *atmospheres* (atm) of gauge pressure:

A. Oxygen cylinder: 2000
B. Nitrous oxide: 750
C. After reducing valves: 3–4
D. Peak inspiratory pressure during IPPV: 0.25
E. PEEP: 0.10.

Answers overleaf

3.1. All correct

1 atmosphere = 760 mmHg
1 mm H_2O = 0.073 mmHg
1 pound/square inch = 51.71 mmHg
1 newton/square metre (Nm^{-2}) = 0.0075 mmHg
1 kilopascal (kPa) = 1 pascal (Pa) $\times$ 10^3
1 pascal = 1 Nm^{-2}
1 kilopascal = 7.501 mmHg
1 mmHg = 0.1333 kPa

Pressure is a measure of force per unit area. One millimetre of water or mercury measures the displacement of either H_2O or Hg up a tube by the pressure being measured. The SI (Système International) units have been developed to reduce the many measurement units to a few with international acceptance. A newton is a measure of force in the SI system (and is equivalent to about 4¾ ounces). The pascal is a measure of pressure and the kilopascal is the unit commonly used in medical practice. One kilopascal is about 1/100 atmosphere.

3.2. C

Familiarity with gas pressures in various units is essential to a safe understanding of the behaviour of gases. The high cylinder pressures of oxygen (130 atm) and nitrous oxide (50 atm) fall in the reducing valve to pressures around 3–4 atm. The peak inspiratory pressure (say 25 cm H_2O or 2.5 kPa) is about 1/40 (0.025) normal atmospheric pressure and PEEP of 10 cm H_2O (1 kPa) is about 0.01 atm. A useful clinical approximation is that:

1 atm (1 bar)
= 1 kg/cm^2
= 1000 cm H_2O
= 100 kPa

Thus a normal ventilator pressure of 20 cm H_2O is readily converted to 2 kPa. (Reducing valves are better designated as pressure regulators).

3.3. When gas flows through a tube:

A. Laminar flow implies that flow is smooth and parallel to the wall of the tube

B. With laminar flow, resistance is directly proportional to the diameter of the tube

C. Above the critical flow rate, turbulent flow results

D. At a constriction, a sharp curve, or a valve, turbulent flow develops

E. When turbulence develops, flow is inversely proportional to the square of the velocity.

3.4. Gas flow measurements can be made by devices of various types with distinctive properties:

A. The rotating bobbin is an example of a constant orifice device

B. The Fleisch pneumotachograph is an example of a variable orifice flow meter

C. Any gas with the same density gives correct readings in a rotating bobbin flowmeter

D. Increased back pressure on a rotating bobbin flowmeter means that, at a given indicated flow, there will be an increased number of molecules passing per minute

E. The pressure of the gas at the narrowest part of a Venturi will decrease.

Answers overleaf

3.3. A, C, D

When flow is laminar, Poiseuille's law applies. It states that the flow is proportional to pressure change along the tube and the fourth power of the radius, and inversely proportional to the length of tube and the viscosity of the fluid.

$$Q \propto \frac{\triangle P \times r^4}{L \times \mu}$$

$\triangle P$ = change in pressure, L = length, μ = viscosity, Q = flowrate, r = radius. Above the gas's critical flow rate, generalized turbulence occurs. Turbulent flow also occurs at constrictions, valves, or orifices. At an orifice the flow rate produced by a given pressure is approximately proportional to the square root of the pressure, the square of the diameter and inversely proportional to the density.

3.4. D, E

The pressure under a rotating bobbin stays constant as the increased flow pushes the bobbin up to a wider diameter (larger orifice). The Fleisch places a fine mesh in the stream, which is effectively a constant orifice. No available gas flow measuring device should be trusted to be accurate with a different gas, although the rotating vane (Wright) performs well and the ionization pneumotachograph ought to be independent of gas composition. Back pressure compresses the gas and lowers a rotating bobbin. At a given reading this means *more molecules* are passing, but in a *smaller volume* per minute, i.e. the meter under-reads if you are interested in the supply of molecules, but over-reads if you required a volume of gas to ventilate carbon dioxide out of the patient. These effects are significant in hyperbaric medicine. The pressure falls in the narrow part of a Venturi tube as the velocity increases.

3.5. Henry's law:

    A. Refers to the effect of volume on the temperature of a gas
    B. States that if pressure is held constant the molecular force of a gas will not change
    C. Refers to the concentration of a dissolved gas in a given solvent
    D. Assumes that the temperature is held constant
    E. Relates concentration of a dissolved gas to the partial pressure of that gas.

3.6. The blood/gas coefficient for an inhalation agent:

    A. Defines the solubility of the agent in blood
    B. Defines the potency of an agent
    C. Is related to potency; the lower the solubility, the greater is the potency
    D. For halothane is 12
    E. For N_2O is 0.47.

3.7. Humidity

    A. Expressed in absolute units relates the amount of water present to the maximum amount possible for that temperature
    B. Expressed in absolute units relates the mass of water vapour per unit volume
    C. Is a measure of the total water content, both vapour and droplets
    D. Expressed in relative units compares the humidity at a certain temperature to absolute zero
    E. In the lungs is usually 95–100% of the maximum possible value.

Answers overleaf

3.5. C, D, E

Henry's law states that the concentration of dissolved gas in a given solvent is directly proportional to the partial pressure of the gas, if the temperature remains constant. This law breaks down when applied to very soluble gases. It does not hold for oxygen in blood because most oxygen is chemically combined to haemoglobin. It *does* hold for nitrogen; therefore when pressure falls, nitrogen tends to bubble out of solution. This occurs when a deep sea diver suddenly rises to the surface and develops the 'bends', the 'itch', the 'chokes', or the 'staggers' as the bubbles form in joints, skin, lungs, or brain respectively.

3.6. A, E

Blood/gas coefficients relate to the relative concentrations of an agent between blood and gas when the two phases are in equilibrium. The higher the number the more soluble it is in blood. Greater solubility means a longer time is necessary to reach equilibrium between the alveolar and the inspired gas tension and therefore the induction of anaesthesia is prolonged. Blood/gas coefficients for some inhalation agents are cyclopropane 0.42, nitrous oxide 0.47, isoflurane 1.41, enflurane 1.78, halothane 2.36, diethyl ether 12.1, and methoxyflurane 13.0. It is *fat* solubility which correlates with potency.

3.7. B, E

The mass of water vapour per unit volume is absolute humidity. The addition of particles (or droplets) of water may change the water content of the air, but it does not raise the humidity beyond 100%. Relative humidity measures the percent of the maximum possible water vapour for the temperature that is actually present:

$$\text{Relative humidity (\%)} = \frac{\text{partial pressure of } H_2O \text{ vapour present}}{\text{saturated vapour pressure at that temperature}} \times 100$$

The relative humidity in the lungs is usually 95–100%. Water vapour is added to inspired air mainly by the nose. If the nose is bypassed, the addition of humidity to the inspired air is provided by the tracheal and bronchial mucous membrane.

3.8. Which oil/gas coefficients are correct:

A. Nitrous oxide—1.4
B. Halothane—422
C. Enflurane—98.5
D. Isoflurane—168
E. Methoxyflurane—64.

3.9. If a gas passes through a container which holds a volatile liquid:

A. The gas will stop flowing when its pressure falls to the vapour pressure of the liquid
B. The gas will not mix with the vapour of the volatile liquid
C. The gas will turn to liquid
D. The mixture of the gas and the vapour will obey Dalton's law of partial pressure
E. Some gas dissolves in the volatile liquid.

3.10. Which is true of an ideal gas?

A. The volume at a given pressure is inversely proportional to its temperature
B. The volume of a gas is directly proportional to its pressure
C. At absolute zero the volume of a gas would be 1 volume per cent
D. One mole of any gas occupies the same volume as 1 mol of any other gas at a given temperature and pressure
E. The ideal gas law is a combination of Boyle's, Charles' and Avogadro's law.

Answers overleaf

3.8. A, C

The oil/gas coefficient is related to potency. The more soluble the agent is in oil, the more potent it is; therefore nitrous oxide with an oil/gas coefficient of 1.4 is relatively weak. Methoxyflurane's oil/gas coefficient is 825 representing a potent agent.

Agents of intermediate potency are halothane: 224, enflurane: 98.5, and isoflurane: 99. The figures represent solubility in olive oil, which is used as the standard *in vitro* solvent.

3.9. D, E

A gas passing through a container which holds a volatile liquid will mix with the vapour of that liquid. The resulting mixture will follow Dalton's law of partial pressure which states that the total pressure of a mixture of gases is equal to the sum of the partial pressures of the individual gases. At atmospheric pressure (760 mmHg), and when the mixture is saturated with halothane at room temperature (241 mmHg at 20°C), the partial pressure of the gas will be 519 mmHg. Some of the gas entering the container dissolves in the volatile liquid. This can be significant if two vaporizers are in sequence and both used at once. The agent in the second vaporizer becomes contaminated by dissolving vapour from the first. Transfilling events are further complicated by condensation when the 'downstream' vaporizer contains liquid of a lower boiling point than the 'upstream' vaporizer.

3.10. D, E

Boyle's law states that the volume of a given quantity of a gas is inversely proportional to its pressure. Charles' law states that, at a constant pressure, the volume of a given quantity of a gas is directly proportional to the absolute temperature. Absolute temperature is measured in degrees kelvin. At absolute zero or 0 K (which is equal to $-273.16°C$), a gas theoretically has *no* volume. Avogadro's law states that 1 mol of any gas occupies the same volume as 1 mol of any other gas at the same temperature and pressure. The ideal gas law is a combination of the above three laws: $PV = nRT$; P = pressure, V = volume, n = the number of molecules of the gas present, R = a constant, T = absolute temperature.

3.11. **A new volatile anaesthetic has a vapour pressure of 190 mmHg. What is the per cent of anaesthetic delivered from a measured flow vaporizer if the total flow is 3 l and the flow to the vaporizer is 300 ml?**

    A. 33%
    B. 3.3%
    C. 2.5%
    D. 0.2%
    E. 1%.

3.12. In clinical practice at sea level:

    A. The vapour pressures of all commonly used anaesthetics equals the atmospheric pressure
    B. The vapour pressures of all commonly used anaesthetics equals their boiling points
    C. The highest partial pressure of a gas that can be achieved at a given temperature is its vapour pressure
    D. The vapour pressure of commonly used anaesthetics varies with the barometric pressure
    E. The vapour pressure of commonly used anaesthetics varies with the temperature.

3.13. Which of the following vapour pressures in mmHg are correct for 20°C?

    A. Halothane, 241
    B. Diethyl ether, 440
    C. Methoxyflurane, 23
    D. Enflurane, 360
    E. Trichlorethylene, 636.

Answers overleaf

3.11. B

The percent concentration of a volatile anaesthetic coming from a measured flow vaporizer can be calculated by the following formula:

$$\frac{(F_V) \left(\dfrac{VP}{(AP - VP)} \right)}{F_t} \times 100 = \% \text{ conc.}$$

F_t = Total gas flow
F_V = Flow to the vaporizer
VP = Vapour pressure
AP = Atmospheric pressure

A useful approximation is as follows: The mixture leaving the vaporizer contains vapour at 190 mmHg (1/4 atmosphere) with oxygen occupying the other 3/4 atmosphere. Thus the 300 ml of oxygen supplied (being 3/4 of the total) must be accompanied by 100 ml of anaesthetic vapour (1/4 of the total); 100 ml of vapour in 3000 ml is about 3.3%. Slightly greater accuracy is obtained by adding into the total flow the oxygen passing through the vaporizer. The final proportion is then 100 ml of vapour in 3300 ml, or approximately 3%.

3.12. C, E

The vapour pressure of different volatile agents depends on the agent and the ambient temperature. Vapour pressure is independent of barometric pressure. The boiling point of a liquid is that temperature at which the vapour pressure is equal to the atmospheric pressure; it therefore varies with atmospheric pressure.

3.13. A, B, C

The vapour pressure at 20°C of enflurane is 175 mmHg, and of trichlorethylene is 60 mmHg.

3.14. The copper kettle:

A. Is a variable bypass vaporizer
B. Is temperature compensated by supplied heat
C. Is made of copper because of its low heat capacity and thermal conductivity
D. When used with low flows and IPPV can deliver higher than predicted concentrations
E. As a low efficiency type it can be used within a closed circuit system.

3.15. The Fluotec Mark II:

A. Is temperature-compensated
B. Should be used with a 4 l/min or greater fresh gas flow
C. If set half the distance between 0% and 0.5% will deliver about 0.45%
D. Is markedly affected by back pressure when fresh gas flows are over 2 l/min.
E. Because of its low internal resistance it can be used as a draw-over vaporizer.

3.16. The Fluotec Mark III:

A. Is an agent-specific, flow-over wick-type vaporizer
B. Lacks a temperature-compensation device
C. At less than 3% delivers relatively reliable concentrations at any fresh gas flow
D. Is designed to function safely even when tipped
E. Has a smaller chamber volume than the Mark II.

Answers overleaf

3.14. B, D

The copper kettle is a measured flow vaporizer (as opposed to a variable bypass type). Copper has a high heat capacity and thermal conductivity. At a total flow of 500 ml/min, an 18 ml/min flow through the kettle should produce 1.8% halothane. However, with IPPV, concentrations of 4–8% have been delivered. This is due to intermittent pressure causing a surging of gas in and out of the vaporizer carrying more vapour. Heat is usually supplied from the room by conduction, but heaters have also been used. Its construction and functional principle determine it as highly efficient and quite unsuitable for insertion within a closed circuit.

3.15. A, B, C

The Fluotec Mark II is temperature-compensated by a bimetallic strip at the outlet. With this model, concentration settings less than 0.5% are not trustworthy. Back pressure affects it significantly when fresh gas flows are less than 2 l/min.

3.16. A, C, E

The Fluotec Mark III is temperature-compensated by a bimetallic strip. Tipping a filled vaporizer can allow liquid halothane to get into the outlet and thereby deliver very high concentrations of halothane. Its improved characteristics over the Mark II are partly related to its lower volume, higher pressure chamber.

Physics

3.17. Which of the following are true?

A. A variable bypass vaporizer is one in which the total flow
of the fresh gas goes to the vaporizer
B. A measured flow vaporizer has a bypass valve which directs
part of the total gas flow through the volatile liquid
C. A draw-over vaporizer is one in which the carrier gas passes
over the surface of the liquid
D. In-circuit vaporizers are incorporated into the patient's
breathing system
E. Out-of-circuit vaporizers must have a low resistance
because high pressure can be generated in their use.

**3.18. A vaporizer for a volatile agent may be in the circuit (VIC) or
it may be in the fresh supply outside the circuit (VOC). Which
of the following combinations would be expected to lower the
inhaled vapour concentration:**

A. VIC, increased fresh gas flow
B. VIC, decreased fresh gas flow
C. VIC, decreased ventilation
D. VOC, decreased fresh gas flow
E. VOC, decreased ventilation

3.19. Which of the following are true:

A. If the diathermy ground is faulty, the current can go
through the anaesthesia machine
B. The chance of burns from a diathermy is increased by using
a small ground pad
C. If the diathermy ground is faulty, burns can occur under
the ECG electrodes
D. The danger of diathermy is decreased by placing the
grounding pad as far away from the operative site as
possible
E. It is hazardous to place the ground pad on the leg below
the knee.

Answers overleaf

87

3.17. A, C, D

In a variable bypass vaporizer the total flow of fresh gas goes to the vaporizer, but only some of this flow comes into contact with the anaesthetic agent; the remainder is bypassed. In a measured flow vaporizer, a known flow of carrier gas is run through the vaporizer. This carrier gas picks up the anaesthetic and then this mixture is introduced to the total gas flow. An example of this type of vaporizer is a copper kettle. It is the in-circuit vaporizers which must have a low resistance to minimize resistance for the patient.

3.18. A, C, D

There is continuous uptake of anaesthetic by the patient (and losses via rubber, etc). This uptake means that when the vaporizer is outside the circuit, the inhaled vapour concentration is lower than that supplied from the vaporizer. However, when the vaporizer is in the circuit, vaporization depends upon ventilation circulating the gas; the inhaled concentration therefore falls if the ventilation falls. The table below shows the effects on inhaled concentration:

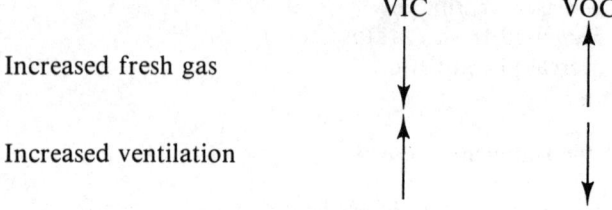

3.19. A, B, C, E

Diathermy is probably the greatest electrical risk faced by the surgical patient today. With a poor ground the current will travel to earth by the shortest possible route. This may be through the anaesthetic machine or the ECG electrodes. A small ground pad would concentrate the current and possibly cause a burn. The knee is a very poor conductor of electricity and so the ground pad should not be placed on the lower leg.

3.20. There may be a difference between the anaesthetic concentration supplied by a machine and that inspired by the patient because of:

A. Rebreathing of exhaled gas
B. The fit of the mask
C. Absorption of the anaesthetic gases by the anaesthetic system
D. Air dilution in open systems
E. Evolution of anaesthetic gases from the anaesthesia system.

3.21. Factors involved in determining brain levels of volatile inhalation anaesthetics are:

A. The altitude at which the anaesthetic is administered
B. The patient's minute ventilation
C. Uptake of the agent from the lungs
D. Passage of the agent across the blood–brain barrier
E. Metabolic rate for the given agent

3.22. The second gas effect:

A. Slows the rate of rise of alveolar concentration of another gas
B. Tends to lead to tissue hypoxia during induction
C. Causes an increase in alveolar ventilation
D. Tends to increase the concentration of the primary agent in the alveoli
E. Persists throughout anaesthesia.

Answers overleaf

3.20. All correct

Rebreathing dilutes the inspired anaesthetic, as does atmospheric air drawn in from under a loose mask. Halogenated hydrocarbons may be absorbed by, or given off from, rubber tubing before reaching the patient.

3.21. B, C, D

The agent must be generated either by vaporization or from a gaseous source in concentration adequate for anaesthesia. At high altitudes, vaporizers continue to produce effective anaesthetic concentrations. As the ambient pressure is less, this effective anaesthetic level is, of course, a larger fraction of the overall pressure. The minute ventilation must be sufficient to deliver the agent to the lungs. As Eger points out (*Anaesthetic Uptake and Action*, p. 133, 1974): 'The lesser uptake which accompanies a lower cardiac output permits a more rapid rise in alveolar anaesthetic partial pressure. However, if the lower output is shared proportionately by all tissues, including the brain, then the reduced cerebral blood flow slows the transfer of the higher alveolar partial pressure to the brain'. Finally the agent must be able to cross the blood–brain barrier.

Metabolism of an inhalation agent may be important in relation to toxic effects, but it plays no role in the initial determination of brain concentrations.

3.22. None correct

During induction the rapid uptake of N_2O from the lungs tends to increase the intake of other gases into the lungs. As N_2O is absorbed there is an increased concentration of *other* agents, including oxygen, this is the second gas effect. The increased gas entering the lungs cannot be regarded as increased ventilation because no carbon dioxide will be carried away. If anything the elimination of carbon dioxide might be temporarily reduced. The effect is largely over after several minutes at which time the rate of body uptake of N_2O begins to decrease towards equilibrium.

3.23. The uptake of anaesthetic agent from the lung:

A. Is increased by greater blood solubility of the agent
B. Is increased by greater cardiac output
C. Is decreased by high venous concentration of the agent
D. Is decreased by high alveolar concentration of the agent
E. Is decreased by high alveolar ventilation.

3.24. The concentration effect describes:

A. The difference between behaviour of real gases and theoretical properties of 'ideal' gases
B. The enhanced uptake of oxygen during nitrous oxide inhalation
C. The enhanced uptake of halothane during nitrous oxide inhalation
D. The enhanced uptake of nitrous oxide during nitrous oxide inhalation
E. The maintenance of the gaseous state when nitrous oxide and oxygen are mixed at high concentrations in the same cylinder.

3.25. A pressure transducer used to measure arterial or venous blood pressures:

A. Is a device which changes electrical current into mechanical motion
B. Typically has a chamber for blood
C. Has a diaphragm and sensor which converts motion to an electrical signal
D. Has sensing elements, such as digital displays and oscilloscopes, in contact with its diaphragm
E. Should have a high compliance.

Answers overleaf

3.23. A, B, C

The higher concentration in the venous blood, the less the gradient between the lung and the blood. When the concentration in the venous blood equals that in the alveoli, uptake stops.

Likewise a high alveolar concentration changes the gradient in favour of greater uptake. This is the rationale for using a concentration of inhalation agents above that needed for surgery during induction. The higher the cardiac output and the alveolar ventilation, the greater the uptake.

3.24. D

When a gas such as nitrous oxide is inhaled at high concentration, its absorption causes a mass inflow to replace the gas taken-up. This inflow hastens the equilibrium between inspired and alveolar partial pressures and tends to shorten induction. The higher the inhaled concentration, the more rapid the rise in alveolar concentration. It is not significant at low concentrations (e.g. with halothane) as absorption results in no appreciable mass inflow. The way that nitrous oxide enhances the absorption of halothane, or oxygen, is referred to as the second-gas effect.

3.25. C

A pressure transducer changes the mechanical force of a fluid into an electrical signal. A chamber filled with fluid (not blood) is in continuity with the artery or vein in which the pressure is being measured. In the base of this chamber is a diaphragm which moves as pressure changes in the system. This movement of the diaphragm is detected by a sensing element in contact with the diaphragm, typically a strain gauge whose resistance is altered. A good pressure transducer has a low compliance so that the volume of fluid required to move the diaphragm is minimal.

3.26. A correctly adjusted calibrated transducer, amplifier and paper chart recorder are used to record blood pressure. An oscilloscope is used to display the same pressure, but requires calibration. A customary sequence of adjustments includes which of the following:

    A. Adjust transducer height to obtain zero on oscilloscope
    B. Open transducer to air and adjust gain control on chart recorder to obtain zero on oscilloscope
    C. Apply known pressure and adjust gain control followed by applying zero pressure and adjusting zero control
    D. First adjust oscilloscope gain control and then oscilloscope zero control
    E. First adjust oscilloscope zero control and then the oscilloscope gain control.

3.27. The peak arterial line pressure measured using a strain gauge, amplifier and cathode ray oscilloscope may under-read or over-read. Which of the following may influence the accuracy of the recorded systolic pressure:

    A. The degree of damping
    B. Catheter length
    C. Compliance of transducer and tubing
    D. The frequency response of the catheter/transducer
    E. The artery selected for line placement.

3.28. Which of the following are true concerning electrodes for blood gas analysis?

    A. The oxygen electrode employs the paramagnetic property of O_2
    B. The oxygen electrode functions because of the reaction:
        $O_2 + 2H_2 \rightarrow 2 H_2O$
    C. The oxygen electrode has a platinum cathode and a silver/silver chloride anode
    D. The carbon dioxide electrode relies on CO_2 diffusing into a solution of bicarbonate
    E. The CO_2 electrode is a modified pH electrode.

Answers overleaf

3.26. E

In general, alteration of the gain control will vary all the scale readings except a correctly adjusted zero. It is therefore customary to first open the transducer to 'zero' pressure (atmospheric) and set the zero control; then when the gain is adjusted it is likely to leave the zero point still correct. As the recorder is set correctly here, the oscilloscope requires the adjustment. The zero is adjusted first, then the gain.

3.27. All correct

All these factors are important. The accurate measurement of systolic pressure requires a system which responds appropriately to rapid variations in pressure. The transducer and catheter must be considered together. Their joint function determines the properties of the system. The degree of damping (D) conveniently incorporates: viscous resistance (R), inertial mass (M), stiffness (S).

$$D = \frac{R}{2\,MS}$$

When there is too little damping (<1) there is overshoot, too much (>1) and the peak is never reached; 0.66 is an excellent compromise allowing rapid response with minimal overshoot. The frequency response of the system should be at least 50% above the highest harmonic, which in the case of blood pressure is about 20 Hz; therefore a 30 Hz response is acceptable. A distal artery in a noncompliant vascular system may give misleadingly high readings. The inertial mass of the blood moving down the stiff vascular system causes over-reading due to under-damping. A distal artery may also give a low reading due to vasoconstriction or stenosis of a proximal artery.

3.28. C, D, E

At the platinum cathode of an O_2 electrode the following reaction takes place $O_2 + 4\,e \rightarrow 2\,O^{--}$. The ionized molecule moves to the silver/silver chloride anode causing a current. The greater the amount of O_2, the greater the current.

The CO_2 electrode is basically a pH electrode. CO_2 travels from the blood, across a Teflon membrane and into a sodium bicarbonate solution. The change in pH caused by the CO_2 is measured.

3.29. Two variables x and y are related as follows: y = 4 x + 5, correlation coefficient (r) = − 0.9:

    A. The slope of this line is 0.25
    B. The x intercept is − 0.8
    C. The y intercept is 20
    D. There is a very good correlation
    E. This correlation coefficient is inappropriate.

3.30. When a variable has a normal distribution:

    A. 32% of the population lie outside ± 1 standard deviation
    B. The standard error measures the scatter of the population
    C. 2.5% of the population exceed + 2 standard deviations
    D. The shape of the distribution curve (bell-shaped) corresponds to the formula of the type: $y = e^{-(x^2)}$
    E. The distribution is also known as Gaussian.

3.31. The following computer terms are appropriately explained as follows:

    A. One byte of information is sufficient to define one of 64 possibilities
    B. Analog data is the type processed by the modern generation of microcomputer
    C. CPU is the abbreviation for Computer's Peripheral Unit.
    D. BASIC is the fundamental machine language that computers use internally
    E. RAM is the abbreviation for reusable address mode
    F. A to D converter turns alternating current (a.c.) to direct current (d.c.).

Answers overleaf

3.29. E

The slope of the line is obtained by considering the effect of increasing the x variable by 1; y rises by 4 and thus the slope is 4. At the y intercept (x = 0) y = (4 × 0) + 5 = 5. At the x intercept (y = 0) 4 x + 5 = 0, x = − 1.25. As the slope has a positive value, so must the correlation coefficient be positive too, thus − 0.9 must be an error.

3.30. A, C, D, E

The standard deviation measures the scatter (variability of the population), the standard error measures the variability of the mean. ± one standard deviation excludes 16% of the population lying above and 16% lying below (total 32%). Similarly two standard deviations exclude a total of 5% (2.5% below and 2.5% above). $y = e^{-(x^2)}$; therefore at x = 0, y = 1. Any negative or positive value of x gives a positive value for x^2 and accordingly a negative value for $-(x^2)$; y therefore reaches a maximum of 1 in the centre and diminishes both sides. The distribution is known as Gaussian.

3.31. None

Microcomputers process digital data, which is a sequence of 'bits' (on/off or one/zero signals). For computers to process a smoothly changing variable, like a voltage or pressure, an analog to digital converter (A to D) is required. Digital data is often processed eight bits (= 1 byte) at a time. Eight bits (one byte) permit $2^8 = 256$ combinations. The manipulation of the data is performed with a central processor unit (CPU) which sends data to and from Random Access Memory (RAM). The fundamental language of computers is the machine code (which varies depending upon the company and product in use). This code is conveniently manipulated by a device called an assembler (using 'assembly language'), or more conveniently still by one of the high level languages (BASIC, FORTRAN, etc) which read (almost) like English.

3.32. A nebulizer:

A. Of the mechanical type relies on a jet of gas blowing water up against a ball
B. Of the mechanical type produce particles of 4 microns or less
C. Of the mechanical type is most efficient at delivering moisture to the lower airway
D. Of the ultrasonic type has a transducer which breaks up the water into particles
E. Of the ultrasonic type produces particles in the 2–5 micron range.

3.33. When a patient is ventilated mechanically with a ventilator attached to a closed circuit, the mechanical dead space:

A. Arises partly from elasticity of the hoses
B. Arises partly from compressibility of the gases
C. Increases as inflation pressure rises
D. Is not altered if a humidifier is added to the circuit
E. Is eliminated when a non-rebreathing valve is inserted in the circle at the Y-piece.

3.34. Relief valves on anaesthetic systems:

A. Are needed because gas flow rates can be greater than patient uptake rates
B. Should open for spontaneous breathing at about 0.05–0.1 kPa (0.5 – 1.0 cm of H_2O)
C. Tend to open at higher pressures in the presence of humidity
D. Of the low-pressure type open at or just above the patients peak expiratory pressure
E. Of the low-pressure type can jam in the sealed position causing a pressure rise in the anaesthetic system.

Answers overleaf

3.32. A, B, D

The mechanical nebulizer functions by blowing water up against a ball and thereby breaking it into particles. Most particles larger than 5 microns 'rain out' into the reservoir or breathing tubing. Most of the particles delivered to the patient are in the 2–4 microns range, though some are as small as 0.1 microns.

The ultrasonic nebulizer consists of a transducer whose vibrating diaphragm produces particles mostly between 0.8 to 1 micron.

A water particle larger than 1.5 microns is likely to 'rain out' in the breathing tube or the upper airway. Because of the efficiency of the ultrasonic nebulizer too much water may be delivered and absorbed. This can result in fluid overload or water intoxication.

3.33. A, B, C

The movement of the bellows is not an accurate measure of tidal volume; compression of the gas and stretching of hoses mean that not all of the tidal volume reaches the patient. These sources of dead space are worse at higher pressures or when the circuit volume is increased (e.g. by a humidifier). A non-rebreathing valve will not eliminate losses due to compressibility and elasticity.

3.34. A, B, C, E

There are two types of relief valve: the high pressure type designed to be set to open at a specific pressure; the low-pressure type designed to open if the rate of pressure rise is slow. The low-pressure type is closed by a rapid rise in pressure, as occurs in assisted or controlled ventilation; it can remain jammed shut if the pressure fails to return to near atmospheric.

3.35. Rebreathing of exhaled gases through an anaesthetic system:

    A. Is undesirable because of the heat loss involved
    B. Increases FIo_2 by adding the exhaled O_2 to the inspired O_2 supplied by the machine
    C. Has little effect on $PaCO_2$ because CO_2 is so much more diffusible than O_2
    D. Prolongs both induction and emergence times
    E. Hastens induction, but prolongs emergence.

3.36. Mapleson described and classified various types of anaesthesia circuits:

    A. He described four circuits A, B, C, D
    B. The Bain is a Mapleson C
    C. The T-piece is a Mapleson D
    D. Used for spontaneous ventilation the Mapleson A will deliver fresh gas to the alveoli only when the fresh gas flow rate equals or exceeds the minute ventilation.
    E. Used for spontaneous ventilation a T-piece circuit requires a fresh gas flow rate of 1.5–2 times the patient's minute ventilation.

3.37. The T-piece system:

    A. Should have reservoir tubing of 1.25 cm diameter if used on adults
    B. Allows no rebreathing
    C. Must be modified in order to control ventilation
    D. Has dead space between the fresh gas inlet and the mask
    E. May allow air dilution.

Answers overleaf

3.35. D

Rebreathing retards heat and water loss from the patient; the FIO_2 tends to decrease somewhat because of dilution by expired gases. Alveolar gas tensions are slower to rise during induction and slower to fall during emergence than if a non-rebreathing system was used.

3.36. E

Mapleson described five circuits. The T-Piece (E) becomes a (D) when a valve and bag are added (Bain). A generous tidal volume with controlled ventilation permits the low fresh gas flow to be employed which Bain recommends (70 ml/kg). This is because the tidal volume employed achieves adequate mixing of gas between the alveoli and the circuit; consequently it is mostly alveolar gas which is lost from the circuit. The Mapleson A circuit is efficient for spontaneous ventilation and delivers fresh gas to the alveoli with fresh gas flow rates as low as the patient's *alveolar* ventilation.

3.37. A, D, E

For children the reservoir tubing should be 1 cm in diameter while for adults it should be 1.25 cm in diameter. Rebreathing depends on the fresh gas flow, the patient's minute volume, whether ventilation is spontaneous or controlled and, to a lesser extent, on whether the inspiratory flow pattern is peaked and the expiratory flow pattern is prolonged with no expiratory pause. Air dilution refers to air inspired via the expiratory limb. If the volume of the expiratory limb is less than the tidal volume, air dilution may occur with spontaneous ventilation depending upon fresh gas flow.

Ventilation may be controlled without modification by occluding the expiratory limb of the T-piece and allowing the fresh gas flow to inflate the lungs. Air dilution will not occur with controlled ventilation.

3.38. The Mapleson D system:

A. Differs from a Mapleson A only in the position of the expiratory valve

B. Differs from a Mapleson B only in the position of the fresh gas inlet

C. Is the only system in the Mapleson classification that does not have a T-piece

D. Allows fresh gas to flow away from the patient during his expiratory pause

E. Can function as a T-piece circuit when the bag and valve are detached

Answers overleaf

3.38. D, E

The Mapleson D system consists of a T-piece with a fresh gas inlet next to the mask adaptor, a reservoir tube connecting the fresh gas inlet to the expiration valve, and a reservoir bag at the most distant end from the fresh gas inlet. The Mapleson B system is identical, except that the expiratory valve is between the fresh gas inlet and the patient tube.

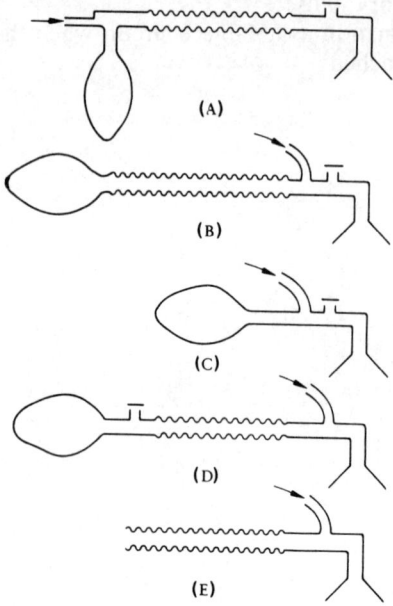

3.39. Which of the following are true about soda lime:

   A. It contains 4% $Ba(OH)_2$ by weight
   B. It contains 14–19% H_2O by weight
   C. Its efficiency increases as its water content increases above 20%
   D. A chemical reaction involved in removal of the patients CO_2 includes $CO_2 + H_2O \leftrightharpoons H_2CO_3$
   E. A chemical reaction involved in removal of the patients CO_2 includes $2\,NaOH + 2\,H_2CO_3 + Ca(OH)_2 \rightleftharpoons Ca\,CO_3 + Na_2CO_3 + 4\,H_2O$

3.40. The main components of resistance in a circle system include:

   A. The flutter valves
   B. The breathing tubes
   C. The CO_2 absorber
   D. The pressure relief valves
   E. The 'T-piece'.

3.41. Which is true of the inspired concentration delivered from a circle system:

   A. Before starting fresh gas flow, the nitrogen concentration is 79%
   B. The nitrogen concentration will no longer be significant after 2 minutes of 2 l of fresh gas flow
   C. A CO_2 of over 6% could occur if both flutter valves leak
   D. The O_2 concentration can be calculated from the fresh gas flow meters if the total flow of $N_2O + O_2$ is greater than 2 l
   E. The O_2 concentration is independent of the uptake of N_2O.

Answers overleaf

3.39. B, D, E

Soda lime by wet weight contains 4% NaOH, 1% KOH, 14–19% H_2O and the remainder is $Ca(OH)_2$ with silicates. Although water is needed for the reaction with carbon dioxide, an excess decreases the efficiency of soda lime and increases the resistance to flow (breathing).

Soda lime particles should be 4–8 mesh in size for optimal activity. Too loose packing in a CO_2 absorber allows channelling, while too tight packing increases the resistance to breathing.

3.40. A, C, D

The flutter valves, CO_2 absorber and pressure relief valves are the main components of increased resistance to breathing in a circle system. However, when extremely low fresh gas flows are used, the pressure relief valve remains closed and offers no resistance to breathing.

The breathing tube has very little influence on total resistance. The length of the tubes can be increased when appropriate without a significant increase in airway resistance.

3.41. A, C, D

Before gas flows are started air will be in the system and therefore the N_2 concentration will start at 79%. With fresh gas flows above 4 l/min, most nitrogen will be gone from the system within 3 minutes. Leaking unidirectional valves (flutter valves) cause rebreathing and high CO_2 concentrations can be obtained. Below 1.2 l/min total fresh gas flow the inspired oxygen concentration cannot be predicted from the N_2O/O_2 ratio set on the flow meters. Nitrous oxide has a second gas effect on oxygen during induction of anaesthesia.

3.42. In a circle system:

  A. Inspiratory gas temperatures range from room temperature to about 32°C
  B. Initial humidity is about 30%
  C. Decreasing the fresh gas flow increases the humidity
  D. The humidity will be reduced when a patient's CO_2 output is small, e.g. in children
  E. Wetting the breathing tubes before use does not change the humidity in the system.

3.43. CO_2 absorbers:

  A. May be designed with two chambers in parallel
  B. May be designed with two chambers in series
  C. May have two separate chambers to allow flow to and from the circle system
  D. May be designed with a tube on the outside to return gas to the circle system
  E. May have a bypass which should be left in the 'on' position when low flow rates (0.5–1 l/min) are used.

Answers overleaf

3.42. A, B, C, D

When a system is first used the humidity is about 30%, this may rise to about 61% after 1½ hours of use because the absorption of CO_2 creates water. If fresh gas flows of 500 ml/min are used 93% humidity can be obtained after a period of use. Wetting the breathing tubes with water does increase the humidity in a circle system.

3.43. A, B, D

Some CO_2 absorbers were designed with two parallel chambers with the intention that one chamber could be regenerating while the other was being used. Most have the chambers in series. Flow through modern CO_2 absorbers is unidirectional, not to and from the circle system. Gas returns either through a side tube or a tube in the centre of the absorber. The side tube is preferred because the central tube may allow channelling to occur around it. Some CO_2 absorbers have a bypass which eliminates the absorber from the system. This is safe at high gas flows, but would allow marked CO_2 retention at low flows.

3.44. Which of the following are true about defibrillators?

A. The appropriate energy to defibrillate an adult is 10 watt/sec

B. Defibrillation works by causing all the cells of the myocardium to depolarize at the time of the shock and then repolarize together

C. To defibrillate a heart, the synchronization unit should be turned on

D. To defibrillate a heart one paddle should be placed on the right upper chest and the other on the left upper chest

E. Both paddles must not be held by the same individual.

3.45. A modern defibrillator designed for ventricular defibrillation or synchronized counter shock:

A. Delivers a short burst of 50 or 60 Hz a.c. current for about 0.2 seconds.

B. Delivers up to about 400 volts d.c.

C. Delivers up to about 400 Joules

D. Is most effective with one paddle to the right of the upper sternum and the other over the apex

E. Can be appropriately tested through a 50 ohm resistance.

Answers overleaf

3.44. B

To defibrillate a heart of an adult patient with a closed chest, the maximum output (400 watt/sec or Joule) of the defibrillating unit should be used. The paddles should be placed anteriorly and posteriorly, or on the upper right chest and the lower left chest (over the apex of the heart). During open heart surgery, when the paddles are applied directly to the heart, a charge of 15–30 watt/sec is adequate. The synchronization unit is turned on when the defibrillator is used for a cardioversion; the unit will then not fire until an R wave is sensed. Conversely in the case of fibrillation, the unit *will not discharge* if the synchronization unit is 'on'. It is safer, but not essential, if each paddle is held by a different individual.

3.45. C, E

The a.c. defibrillators have almost disappeared. The d.c. defibrillator stores a charge, up to about 400 watt/sec (Joules), some or most of which is discharged to the patient. (New models may indicate charge delivered rather than charge stored.) The most effective, though less convenient, paddle placement is anterior and posterior. An appropriate load to use for testing defibrillators is 50 ohms.

4. ANATOMY

4.1. The following vertebral levels correspond to the structures shown:

A. C3 body—tip of the epiglottis
B. C4 body— the body of the hyoid bone
C. Top of C5—the vocal cords
D. C5 body—the thyroid cartilage
E. C6 body—first tracheal ring.

4.2. The carina in a normal erect adult:

A. Is about 10 cm from the cricoid cartilage
B. Is at the level of the xiphisternum
C. Is at the level of upper border of T7
D. Rises on deep inspiration by up to 2.5 cm
E. Is about 2.5 cm from the left upper lobe bronchus.

4.3. Which of the following are true about the human nose:

A. Resistance to breathing is half of that through the mouth
B. Its most important function is warming and humidifying inspired air
C. Nasal mucosa is innervated by facial nerve
D. Humidity is provided by secretion from nasal mast cells
E. At room temperature saturated air contains about 2 volumes per cent of water; at body temperature full saturation requires 6 volumes per cent.

Answers overleaf

4.1. A, B, D, E

The vocal cords lie at the level of, and are attached to, the thyroid and arytenoid cartilages. The length/tension of the vocal cords depends upon relative movements of the cricoid, arytenoid and thyroid cartilages under the influence of the cricothyroid and thyro-arytenoid muscle. The correctly positioned endotracheal cuff will normally be no higher than about the body of C6 (the cuff can usually be palpated just below the cricoid if it is inflated and deflated).

4.2. A

Radiographic recognition of correct tracheal and bronchial tube placement depends on familiarity with the anatomy. The carina is at the top of T5, at the angle of Louis, about 10 cm from the cricoid cartilage, 2.5 cm from the right upper lobe bronchus and 5 cm from the left upper lobe bronchus. The carina descends by up to 2.5 cm on deep inspiration.

4.3. B, E

The resistance to breathing through the nose is about 1½ times greater than through the mouth. The nose, with its stiff hairs and spongy mucosa, tends to protect the respiratory tree from foreign particles. Its most important function is the warming and humidification of inspired air. Inhaled air is warmed to about 37° by the time it reaches the larynx and is almost fully saturated with water. Water is added by the secretions of goblet cells and transudates from the mucosa.

Sensory innervation of the mucosa is by the first and second divisions of the trigeminal nerve. Parasympathetic fibres to the blood supply run through branches of the facial nerve while sympathetic innervation comes from a plexus in the area of the internal carotid artery. Stellate ganglion block causes nasal stuffiness due to vasodilation.

4.4. The pharynx obtains motor and sensory innervation as follows:

    A. Sensory fibres from the lesser palatine branch of the vagus (X)

    B. Sensory fibres from the mandibular division of the trigeminal (V)

    C. Sensory fibres from the cranial accessory nerve (XI)

    D. Secretomotor fibres from the stellate ganglion

    E. Motor fibres from the maxillary division of the trigeminal (V).

4.5. The laryngeal muscles receive innervation from the following nerves:

    A. The internal laryngeal

    B. The spinal accessory

    C. The glossopharyngeal

    D. The recurrent laryngeal

    E. The hypoglossal.

4.6. The following vocal cord positions are characteristic:

    A. Cadaveric—the cords are touching

    B. Total paralysis—the cords are touching

    C. Bilateral division of recurrent laryngeal nerves—wide abduction

    D. Partial recurrent laryngeal nerve damage—moderate abduction

    E. Division of left recurrent laryngeal—deviation to the left during phonation.

Answers overleaf

4.4. None correct

The lesser palatine is a branch of the (purely sensory) maxillary division of the trigeminal (V) and supplies the soft palate and tonsil. The motor root of the trigeminal is distributed via the mandibular division and innervates the tensor palati. The cranial accessory (XI) provides motor fibres to the soft palate (except tensor palati). The glossopharyngeal (IX) provides motor fibres to the stylopharyngeus, the vagus (X) to other muscles and both nerves provide secretomotor fibres. The glossopharyngeal also provides sensory fibres for the pharynx and carries taste from the posterior third of the tongue. The gag reflex can be suppressed by blocking the glossopharyngeal.

4.5. D

The only laryngeal muscles not supplied by the recurrent laryngeal branches of the vagus are the cricothyroids supplied by the external laryngeal nerve of the superior laryngeal branch of the vagus. The internal laryngeal nerve is sensory above the vocal cords. The spinal accessory, glossopharyngeal and hypoglossal provide no laryngeal innervation. The spinal accessory innervates the sternomastoid and trapezius; the hypoglossal is the motor nerve of the tongue and the glossopharyngeal provides motor and sensory fibres above the larynx.

4.6. E

The anaesthetist is most familiar with the position of the cords when the patient is totally paralyzed (after suxamethonium for intubation). This is similar to the cadaveric position; the cords are then not tensed by the cricothyroids and lie abducted. Total division of the recurrent laryngeal nerves leaves the cords near the midline, because of preserved tone of the cricothyroid muscles, but with a moderate airway. Division of one nerve prevents abduction during phonation so that the opposing cord moves over beyond the midline. Partial recurrent laryngeal palsy is potentially the most dangerous because the adductor strength is often well maintained and tends to close the airway completely.

4.7. The trachea in an average adult:

- **A.** Is 3–4 cm in diameter
- **B.** Can stretch by up to 2.5 cm during deep inspiration
- **C.** Lies in front of the ascending aorta
- **D.** Is supported by 12 cartilaginous rings
- **E.** Descends almost parallel to the body of the sternum.

4.8. In the normal bronchial tree:

- **A.** The right upper lobe bronchus divides into two after about 4 cm
- **B.** The right lower lobe bronchus gives no medial basal branch
- **C.** The right middle lobe branch is directed posteriorly
- **D.** The left upper lobe branch arises 5 cm from the carina
- **E.** The left and right main bronchi are angled symmetrically in neonates, about 55° from the vertical.

4.9. The blood supply to and from the bronchi has the following characteristics:

- **A.** The bronchial arteries arise from the ascending aorta
- **B.** The bronchial veins deliver blood back directly to the left atrium
- **C.** The bronchial arteries are end arteries and do not anastomose
- **D.** The bronchial veins receive back more blood than delivered by the bronchial artery
- **E.** Bronchial arteries, like pulmonary arteries, show hypoxic vasoconstriction.

4.10. The accessory muscles of respiration include:

- **A.** Sternomastoid
- **B.** Scalenus anterior
- **C.** Scalenus medius
- **D.** Scalenus posterior
- **E.** Intercostals.

Answers overleaf

4.7. B

The trachea is slightly flattened posteriorly and is 1.5–2 cm in transverse diameter. It lies behind the aorta and has 16–20 rings. As it descends it creates an angle with the sternum of about 30°. Not only is it elongated during deep inspiration but, like the bronchi, it also increases in diameter.

4.8. D, E

The right upper lobe bronchus arises about 2.5 cm from the carina and splits after about 1 cm into three segmental bronchi. The right middle lobe bronchus is directed anterolaterally. There is a medial basal segment on the right (but not on the left where the heart is). The left main bronchus is twice as long as the right main and, in adults, is angled 45° (compared with 25° on the right). In neonates the bronchi spread symmetrically at 110° (55° each).

4.9. None correct

The bronchial circulation arises from the descending aorta to supply arterial blood to the bronchi. There is free anastomosis with the pulmonary circulation and some desaturated blood returns in the pulmonary veins to the left atrium; this is one of the anatomic contributions to pulmonary shunting. The bronchial veins therefore receive less blood back and deliver it to the azygos system or sometimes, on the left, to the superior intercostal vein.

4.10. A, B, C, D

The scalene muscles, particularly medius, are active even in quiet ventilation. The sternomastoid is reserved for maximal inspiratory effort. The role of the intercostals in ventilation is complex because activity varies with the phase of ventilation and with segmental height. They are active during speech, as well as during quiet ventilation, and are regarded as primary muscles of ventilation.

4.11. The diaphragm:

A. Is the muscle of respiration that produces about 50% of the normal tidal volume

B. Moves upward and downward about 1.5 cm during quiet respiration

C. Has its range of motion markedly increased by changing from the supine to the sitting position

D. Is weakened sufficiently by unilateral phrenic nerve paralysis to produce a 20% reduction in the maximum breathing capacity

E. Produces 90% of the tidal volume during deep breathing.

4.12. As a molecule of oxygen passes from the alveolus to the pulmonary capillary it passes through:

A. A distance of 2 mm

B. A thin alveolar fluid layer

C. Alveolar epithelial cells

D. The interstitial space

E. The pores of Kohn.

4.13. In the normal cardiac conducting system:

A. The sinoatrial node is a small collection of specialized myocardial tissue located at the junction of the right atrium and the superior vena cava

B. The atrioventricular node is located in the apex of the right ventricle

C. The atrioventricular bundle of His carries impulses from the atrioventricular node to the right and left bundles

D. Fibres of the bundle of His and the origins of the right and left bundle are located in the interventricular septum

E. The right bundle divides into the anterior superior and the posterior inferior fascicles.

Answers overleaf

4.11. B, D

During quiet breathing the 1.5 cm excursion of the diaphragm produce nearly 100% of the tidal volume. The range of motion of the diaphragm does not change when going from the lying to the sitting position. However, the resting level of the diaphragm is high in the lying position due to upward displacement by abdominal contents. During deep breathing, 75% of the tidal volume is produced by the diaphragm and 25% by the intercostals and accessory muscles.

4.12. B, C, D

The gas in the alveoli is separated from the pulmonary blood by a distance of 1–2 microns. Surfactant lines the alveoli. Alveolar epithelium contains three cell types; type I makes up the majority; type II produce the surfactant, and type III are the so-called alveolar brush cells. The interstitial space lies between the epithelial cells and the capillary.

The pores of Kohn connect alveoli allowing gas to travel from one alveolus to another (collateral ventilation).

4.13. A, C, D

Normally the pacemaker of the heart is the sinoatrial node in the right atrium. Impulses travel from it to the atrioventricular node located on the septal wall of the right atrium above the opening of the coronary sinus. From here impulses travel in the bundle of His which divides into the left and right bundle in the interventricular septum. It is the *left* bundle that divides into separate fascicles. Trifascicular heart block (L. anterior, L. posterior and Right) interrupts the entire conducting system and the patient then normally requires an artificial pacemaker.

4.14. Which of the following are true concerning the circulation of the heart:

    A. The right coronary artery arises from the common coronary artery

    B. The right coronary supplies only the right ventricle

    C. The left coronary artery ends as the coronary sinus

    D. The circumflex branch of the right coronary artery circles towards the back of the heart

    E. The left anterior descending branch supplies both ventricles and the interventricular septum.

4.15. In the normal cerebral arterial supply:

    A. The common carotid artery divides into the internal carotid and the vertebral arteries

    B. The right and left vertebral arteries join to form the single basilar artery

    C. The circle of Willis obtains its arterial supply from the anterior and posterior communicating arteries

    D. The anterior inferior cerebellar artery is a branch of the circle of Willis

    E. The middle cerebral artery is a branch of the circle of Willis.

4.16. The respiratory centre of the brain:

    A. Receives impulses from the carotid sinus

    B. Receives impulses via the vagus nerve

    C. Consists of diffusely arranged cells of the reticular formation in the pons

    D. Sends impulses to lower motor neurons via the reticulospinal fibres

    E. Sends impulses to lower motor neurons affecting the diaphragm.

Answers overleaf

4.14. E

The right coronary artery arises from the right aortic sinus. It supplies a branch to the sinoatrial node, a marginal branch to the diaphragmatic surface of the heart, and ends in the posterior descending branch which supplies *both* ventricles posteriorly.

The left coronary artery arises from the left aortic sinus. It divides into the anterior descending, which supplies both ventricles and the interventricular septum, and the circumflex branch which gives off a marginal branch to supply the left ventricle laterally.

Venous drainage is via the coronary sinus system and the anterior cardiac veins which empty into the right atrium. The *smallest cardiac veins* (Thebesian) are minute channels which empty directly into all chambers of the heart. The veins going to the left side of the heart contribute to venous admixture (anatomic shunting).

4.15. B, E

The vertebral arteries originate from the subclavian arteries and combine at the level of the pons to form *one* basilar artery. The two carotids and one basilar supply the circle of Willis. The posterior communicating arteries extend from the posterior cerebral artery forward to anastomose with the ends of the carotids. The anterior cerebral arteries extend forward from the carotid and are joined together by a short anterior communicating artery. The middle cerebral artery is the terminal branch of the internal carotid, while both the anterior and posterior inferior cerebellar arteries are branches of the vertebrals. When internal carotid flow is interrupted during surgery, the pressure in, or back flow from, the upper stump is dependent on the circle of Willis anastomosis.

4.16. B, D, E

The respiratory centre receives impulses from chemoreceptors in the carotid *body*, which monitor PaO_2. Impulses travel to the respiratory centre from the carotid body via the ninth cranial nerve and from the aortic body via the tenth. The respiratory centre, located in the *medulla* consists of reticular formation cells. Efferent impulses travel via reticulospinal fibres to lower motor neurons of the phrenic and intercostal nerves. The respiratory centre also receives impulses via the vagus from the stretch receptors in the lungs and from central chemoreceptors in the floor of the fourth ventricle which respond to local hydrogen ion concentrations.

4.17. Cerebrospinal fluid (CSF):

A. Is produced only in the fourth ventricle
B. Passes anteriorly from the fourth to the third ventricle via the interventricular foramen
C. Is reabsorbed in the lateral ventricles
D. In an adult has a volume of about 300 ml
E. Passes through the dura via the cisterna magna.

4.18. Which of the following is true concerning the blood supply of the spinal cord?

A. There is no anastomosis of spinal arteries, thus the cord is divided into independent vascular areas
B. The two anterior spinal arteries originate from the aorta
C. The two posterior spinal arteries originate from the posterior inferior cerebellar arteries
D. The anterior spinal artery supplies the anterior and lateral columns of the spinal cord
E. The posterior spinal artery supplies the posterior and lateral columns of the cord.

Answers overleaf

4.17. None correct

A normal adult has a CSF volume of about 135 ml; 35 ml in the ventricles, 25 ml in the intracranial subarachnoid space and 75 ml surrounding the spinal cord. Cerebrospinal fluid is formed by the choroid plexuses, which are found mainly in the lateral ventricles, and also in roofs of the third and fourth ventricles. It passes from the lateral ventricles to the third ventricle by the interventricular foramina (of Monro). It reaches the fourth ventricle through the cerebral aqueduct (of Sylvius), which is the narrowest structure through which it must pass. CSF leaves the fourth ventricle via three openings in its roof (the two foramina of Luschka and the median aperture of Magendie) to reach the subarachnoid space around the brain and spinal cord. The cisterna magna is a pocket of CSF in the subarachnoid space between the inferior surface of the cerebellum and the medulla. CSF is reabsorbed by the arachnoid villi and by spinal veins.

4.18. A, C, D

There are two posterior spinal arteries which originate from the posterior inferior cerebellar arteries and run down each side of the cord supplying the posterior columns only. There is only *one* anterior spinal artery which originates at the vertebral arteries and receive communications from the lumbar and intercostal arteries. It runs down the cord in the anterior medial fissure in the pia mater. There is no anastomosis between any of the three arteries and so there are three independent vascular areas of the spinal cord. The anterior spinal artery supplies the anterior and lateral column. Thrombosis of this artery produces the 'anterior spinal artery syndrome', i.e. paraplegia and loss of pain and temperature perception *without* loss of posterior column function (joint position, touch and vibration sensation).

19. The epidural space:

A. Is continuous from inside the skull to its caudal boundary
B. Contains veins which act as collaterals when venous return via inferior vena cava is partially or completely obstructed
C. Is bounded anteriorly by the arachnoid mater
D. Ends caudally at the sacrococcygeal membrane
E. Has an abundant arterial blood supply.

20. In the autonomic nervous system:

A. Sympathetic fibres originate in the cranial nerves and lumbar spinal cord
B. Parasympathetic fibres originate in the thoracic and sacral spinal cord
C. The ganglia of the sympathetic system are located at the end organ
D. The ganglia of the parasympathetic system are located in the paravertebral chain
E. Some sympathetic fibres converge from several levels and pass through the sympathetic chain to form large ganglia.

21. Section (or block with a local anaesthetic) of the stellate ganglion produces:

A. Dilation of the pupil
B. Ptosis of the eyelid
C. Exophthalmus
D. Sweating of the face
E. Vasodilation of the hand.

Answers overleaf

121

4.19. B, D

The epidural space begins at the base of the skull where the dura fuses with the periosteum of the skull. Caudally it ends at the sacrococcygeal membrane. Posteriorly it is bound by the *ligamentum flavum*. Anteriorly it is bound by the dura mater. It has a poor arterial but a rich venous blood supply; these veins provide a collateral return to the heart when the vena cava is obstructed (either partially, as in pregnancy, or completely as the result of a surgical procedure). When acting as collaterals they can become engorged, decreasing the volume of the space and making penetration with an epidural needle more likely. The decrease in volume may cause epidural anaesthesia to reach higher than predicted for the particular dose and volume injected.

4.20. E

The fibres of the sympathetic nervous system originate in the thoracic and lumbar spinal cord (T1–L2). The parasympathetic fibres originate with the cranial nerves (III, VII, IX, X, XI) and from the sacral cord (S2–4). There is a long paravertebral chain of sympathetic ganglia. However, some fibres pass through this paravertebral chain and synapse in large ganglia such as the cervical ganglia, coeliac ganglion and pelvic sympathetic ganglia. Presynaptic parasympathetic fibres usually synapse at the site of their end organs.

4.21. B, E

Sectioning (or blocking with local anaesthetic) of the stellate ganglion produces a Horner's syndrome. The features of a Horner's syndrome are myosis (constriction of the pupil), enophthalmos and ptosis of the eyelid. In addition sweating stops and, therefore, the face and upper extremity feel dry. Vasodilation appears in the vessels of the upper extremity, and in the nose and mouth, giving a feeling of stuffiness.

4.22. Which of the following are true about uterine innervation?

A. Motor activity is primarily a function of the sympathetic nervous system

B. Sympathetic stimulation in the uterus releases acetylcholine as well as noradrenaline

C. Pain sensation of the first stage of labour is carried via afferent sympathetic nerves

D. Pain carrying afferents from the uterus enter the cord at T11 and T12

E. Pain carrying afferents from the vagina enter the cord at L1–3.

4.23. The carotid sinus:

A. Is located just inside the skull in the wall of the internal carotid artery

B. Is primarily a chemoreceptor organ

C. Transmits afferent impulses which travel along the ninth cranial nerve to the medulla

D. Stimulates the medulla to transmit efferent impulses which travel along the tenth cranial nerve.

4.24. Which of the following changes take place in the fetal circulation following birth:

A. Blood flow via the umbilical artery ceases, causing an increase in systemic vascular resistance

B. With the onset of breathing, inflation of the lungs causes an increase in pulmonary vascular resistance

C. The foramen ovale closes because left atrial pressure exceeds right atrial pressure

D. Increased vascular resistance in the lungs causes the ductus arteriosus to close

E. Increase in the newborn's PaO_2 cause constriction of the ductus arteriosus.

Answers overleaf

4.22. A, B, C, D

The parasympathetic nervous system appears to play little part in the motor function of the uterus. However, acetylcholine is released as a *sympathetic* neurotransmitter in the uterus. Pain sensation of uterine contraction and cervical dilation travel along sympathetic afferents to enter the cord at T11 and T12. Pain originating below the cervix travels via afferents which enter the cord at the S2–4 level.

4.23. C, D

The carotid sinus is located at the bifurcation of the common carotid artery. It is primarily a baroreceptor organ which senses changes in blood pressure. A change in blood pressure alters the afferent impulses travelling along the ninth cranial nerve to the vasomotor centre. The efferent impulses travel down the tenth cranial nerve to slow the heart.

4.24. A, C, E

When the umbilical cord is clamped, flow through the umbilical artery to the placenta stops. This eliminates the placenta, which is a low resistance system, and causes the newborn's systemic vascular resistance to rise. Inflation of the lungs converts the pulmonary vascular system into a *low* resistance system. These changes in resistance of the pulmonary and systemic vascular system cause left heart and systemic pressure to rise, while right heart and pulmonary pressure falls. The increase of left atrial pressure above the right atrial pressure causes functional closure of the foramen ovale. Because of the rise in systemic vascular resistance, and the fall in pulmonary vascular resistance, the flow through the ductus arterious should reverse to flow from the aorta to the pulmonary artery. This reverse flow usually does not occur because the increase in the newborn's PaO_2 causes the ductus arteriosus to constrict achieving functional closure shortly after birth. Anatomic closure takes 2–3 weeks.

4.25. Which of the following structural relationships are correct for the stellate ganglion?

    A. The stellate ganglion lies anterior to the transverse process of the seventh cervical vertebra

    B. The stellate ganglion lies anterior to the carotid artery

    C. The phrenic nerve is lateral to the stellate ganglion

    D. The level of the stellate ganglion is inferior to the cricoid cartilage

    E. The level of the stellate ganglion is superior to Chassaignac's tubercle.

4.26. Section (or block with a local anaesthetic) at the level of the axilla of the:

    A. Radial nerve will produce loss of sensation in the lateral portion of the dorsal aspect of the hand and arm

    B. Ulnar nerve will produce loss of sensation in the medial portion of both the dorsal and ventral aspects of the hand

    C. Median nerve will produce loss of sensation in the medial portion of both the dorsal and ventral aspects of the hand

    D. Musculocutaneous nerve will produce loss of sensation in the medial portion of both the dorsal and ventral aspects of the hand

    E. Intercostobrachial nerve will produce loss of sensation in the lateral aspect of the upper arm.

4.27. Components of the brachial plexus:

    A. Pass between the posterior and middle scalene muscles

    B. Are joined by the subclavian artery as it passes in front of the anterior scalene muscle

    C. Pass over the first rib

    D. Are invested in a fascial sheath that originates at the cervical spines and ends slightly beyond the axilla

    E. Innervate the shoulder and arm.

Answers overleaf

Anatomy

4.25. A, C, D

The stellate ganglion lies on the anterior aspect of the transverse process of C7 and the neck of the first rib. The carotid sheath is *anterior* to the stellate ganglion. The phrenic nerve, which lies on the surface of the anterior scalene muscle, is lateral to the stellate ganglion. Overflow of local anaesthetic solution can block the phrenic nerve and/or the recurrent laryngeal branch of the vagus, which is also in close proximity to the stellate ganglion. The stellate ganglion lies just below Chassaignac's tubercle, which is the transverse process of C6.

4.26. A, B

In the anatomic position, the palm of the hand is ventral and the thumb is lateral. The radial nerve provides sensory innervation to the lateral aspect of the lower arm and hand, the ulnar nerve to both the dorsal and ventral aspects of the medial portion of the hand. The median nerve innervates dorsal and ventral aspects of the *lateral* portion of the hand. The musculocutaneous nerve innervates both dorsal and ventral aspects of the lateral part of the forearm. The intercostobrachial nerve is not part of the brachial plexus but arises independently from spinal segment T2. It must be blocked separately from the brachial plexus. It innervates the medial aspect of the upper arm.

4.27. C, D, E

The components of the brachial plexus arise from the anterior rami of C5–T1. They are invested in a continuous fascial sheath as they pass between the anterior and middle scalene muscles, over the first rib, to their termination just below the axilla. The subclavian artery also passes between the anterior and middle scalenes. It is the subclavian vein which passes in front of the anterior scalene muscle. The brachial plexus provides innervation to the shoulder and arm as well as the hand.

Anatomy

4.28. Which of the following are true:

   A. The spinal cord ends at T10
   B. The subarachnoid space ends at S5
   C. The dermatome level of the ventral subcostal margins is T8
   D. The dermatome level of the nipples is T2
   E. The dermatome level of the lateral aspect of the elbow is C5.

4.29. As a needle passes through the midline of the back from the skin into the subarachnoid space, it penetrates which of the following:

   A. The epidural space
   B. The pia mater
   C. The ligamentum teres
   D. The ligamentum flavum
   E. The inferior spinal ligament.

Answers overleaf

127

Anatomy

4.28. C, E

In the adult the subarachnoid space usually ends at S2 and the spinal cord at L1. The commonly used landmarks for determining the height of a spinal anaesthetic are the inguinal ligament T12, the umbilicus T10, the subcostal margin T8, the xiphisternum T6, the nipples T4, the clavicle T2, the medial aspect of the hand C8, the lateral aspect of the hand C6, the lateral aspect of the elbow C5 (the medial aspect is T1), the side of the neck is C3 and the scalp is C2.

4.29. A, D

The tissues in the direct midline from the skin of the back to the subarachnoid space are the skin, subcutaneous tissue, the supraspinous ligament, interspinous ligament, the *ligamentum flavum*, the epidural space, the dura and arachnoid mater. The pia mater is applied directly to the cord itself and is not (normally) penetrated. An epidural needle should, of course, stop short of penetrating any of the meninges.

5. MEDICINE

5.1. Management of a patient with hypothyroidism would include:

A. ECG
B. Starting oral thyroxine at a dose of 0.3 mg/day orally
C. Serum T_3, T_4 and thyroid stimulating hormone (TSH) levels
D. Ruling out secondary hypothyroidism before starting treatment
E. Serum cholesterol estimation.

5.2. Signs of hypothyroidism may include:

A. Brisk ankle jerk
B. Periorbital puffiness
C. Loss of hair
D. Malar flush
E. Thinning of lateral third of the eyebrows.

5.3. Pancreatitis may be associated with:

A. Methaemalbumin
B. Hypercalcaemia
C. Alcoholism
D. Cholelithiasis
E. Polyarteritis nodosa.

Answers overleaf

5.1. A, C, D, E

The heart is often affected by hypothyroidism and the ECG shows a low voltage and sinus bradycardia. There is also a higher incidence of ischaemic heart disease in hypothyroid patients, possibly associated with the raised serum cholesterol levels that are nearly always present with significant hypothyroidism. Immediate treatment of hypothyroidism, especially with high doses of thyroxine, may precipitate myocardial infarction in the patient with concurrent ischaemic heart disease.

Hormonal levels should be determined before instituting thyroxine treatment, beginning with a low dose of 0.025 mg or 0.05 mg daily.

A careful, detailed history may indicate secondary hypothyroidism, in which case immediate treatment with thyroxine may be harmful if pituitary disease is the primary cause.

5.2. B, C, D, E

The relaxation phase of the ankle jerk may be prolonged in hypothyroidism. Thinning of the lateral third of the eyebrows is not always a reliable sign in itself but, in conjunction with other positive signs, is relevant. Periorbital thickening is a characteristic component of the myxoedematous state.

5.3. A, C, D, E

The presence of methaemalbumin in the blood indicates a haemorrhagic necrosis of the pancreas, and the prognosis is poor. Hypocalcaemia is also a cause for concern as the patient with pancreatitis, whose calcium falls below 1·7 mmol/l, often succumbs in spite of calcium replacement. Recurrent attacks of pancreatitis are often a feature of chronic alcoholism.

The relationship between cholelithiasis and pancreatitis is possibly due to the loss of the safety valve effect of the normally distensible gallbladder. This loss allows a rapid rise in biliary pressure in the biliary tract and regurgitation along the pancreatic duct. Polyarteritis nodosa may cause pancreatitis due to local infarction (this is also thought to be the mechanism for pancreatitis in malignant hypertension).

5.4. Management of patients with suspected cerebrovascular disease may include:

   A. EEG
   B. Carotid angiography as a baseline investigation
   C. Computerized axial tomography
   D. Aspirin
   E. Echoencephalography.

5.5. An increased risk of developing atherosclerotic cerebrovascular disease is associated with the following factors:

   A. Abnormal glucose tolerance test
   B. Hypertension
   C. Lipid abnormalities over the age of 55 years
   D. Positive family history
   E. Polycythaemia.

5.6. Anorexia nervosa:

   A. Has a better prognosis in males than in females
   B. Is more common in males
   C. Is easier to control when some other member of the family has a nutritional disorder
   D. Often resolves after marriage
   E. Responds well to insulin therapy.

Answers overleaf

5.4. A, C, D, E

Serial EEGs may be useful in both isolating a lesion and also in distinguishing cerebrovascular disease from a tumour. If initial symptoms are due to an area of infarction secondary to cerebrovascular disease, the EEG will show gradual improvement; with a tumour it will not.

Carotid angiography is an invasive procedure, and may be hazardous to the patient with already compromised cerebral blood flow. The carotid arteries themselves are often the site of significant vascular disease, and an atherosclerotic plaque may be displaced in carrying out the procedure. Thus carotid angiography should be done only when the benefit outweighs the not inconsiderable risk attached to it.

The computerized axial tomography (CAT scan) readily distinguishes between cerebral tumour, abscess, haemorrhage and infarction. Echoencephalography is useful in determining any midline shift and resolution to the shift.

Aspirin and other anticoagulants have been shown to be useful in the medical treatment of cerebrovascular disease.

5.5. A, B, D, E

Lipid abnormalities show an increased risk under the age of 55 years. Other factors that show an increased risk include cardiac impairment, smoking and coronary heart disease. Diabetes mellitus also increases the risk. A positive family history constitutes an important risk factor. Coincidental peripheral arterial disease is present in 30% of patients with cerebrovascular disease.

5.6. None correct

Males are more resistant to developing anorexia nervosa but, when they do, either in association with premorbid obesity and/or major gender identity problems, they do less well than their female counterparts.

Marriage only tends to institutionalize the disorder as the illness is brought to the marriage, whose stability is dependent on the illness continuing.

Both insulin therapy and operant training have low longterm success rates.

7. Acute porphyrias:

A. Are inherited as autosomal recessive traits
B. Often present with abdominal pain and minimal signs
C. Show symptoms attributable to the dysfunction of the autonomic nervous system
D. May have attacks precipitated by ingestion of ethanol
E. May necessitate IPPV during an acute attack.

8. Hyperlipoproteinaemia:

A. Should be screened for in anyone developing coronary heart disease before the age of 55 years
B. Should be treated because this will reverse atherosclerosis
C. Should be treated as a precaution against pancreatitis
D. Type IV is the commonest form associated with coronary heart disease and peripheral vascular disease
E. Is not significantly affected by diet.

Answers overleaf

5.7. B, C, D, E

The acute porphyrias (acute intermittent porphyria, hereditary porphyria and variegate porphyria) are autosomal dominant. The symptoms of an acute attack are attributable to somatic, central and autonomic nervous system dysfunction. Treatment can include IPPV, anticonvulsants, antiemetics, analgesics, β-blocking agents and neostigmine (for severe constipation). Many drugs may precipitate an attack, with barbiturates and oral contraceptives being the most common. Hormonal factors are also important, with attacks occurring more commonly in females during pregnancy and during the week prior to menstruation.

5.8. A, B, C, D

The Joint Working Party for the Royal College of Physicians and the British Cardiac Society suggest screening for hyperlipoproteinaemia in the following groups:

—persons developing coronary heart disease (CHD) or peripheral vascular disease before the age of 55 years
—persons with a strong family history of CHD
—first degree relatives of patients with familial hypercholesterolaemia
—patients with other risk factors such as hypertension, smoking and diabetes mellitus.

Treatment of hypercholesterolaemia has not been shown to reverse atherosclerosis in man, although many studies suggest that it may do so. The treatment of hyperlipoproteinaemia will reverse cutaneous xanthomata, aid in preventing acute pancreatitis and prevent and/or reverse atherosclerosis. It should be treated in a lipid clinic where treatment consists of regularizing the serum lipoproteins by a combination of diet, drug therapy in some cases, and eliminating risk factors such as hypertension, smoking and the use of high oestrogen oral contraceptive preparations.

5.9. **A 50-year-old woman presents to her general practitioner complaining of cold intolerance, lethargy and slowness. On examination her skin is rather dry and coarse; she also has a pulse rate of 56/min. Other relevant symptoms would include:**

- **A.** Menorrhagia
- **B.** Weight gain
- **C.** Flushing and palpitations
- **D.** Paraesthesiae
- **E.** Hoarse voice.

5.10. **Signs and symptoms of a pulmonary embolism may include:**

- **A.** Increased Paco$_2$
- **B.** Rightward shift of the ECG axis with Q_3, T_3 and RSR$'$ patterns in V_1 and V_2
- **C.** Pleural rub, with or without pleural pain
- **D.** Decreased respiratory rate
- **E.** Fever.

5.11. **The following disorders of conduction are best treated by permanent pacemaker implantation:**

- **A.** Asymptomatic bifasicular block
- **B.** Second degree A–V block
- **C.** Sinus arrest
- **D.** Asymptomatic complete A–V block
- **E.** Wolff–Parkinson–White syndrome.

Answers overleaf

5.9. A, B, D, E

Although the symptoms of hypothyroidism and the menopause may be similar in some aspects, a pulse rate of 56/min would indicate that this lady is probably hypothyroid, and flushing and palpatations would not be relevant.

Other symptoms of hypothyroidism include poor memory, constipation and loss of sweating.

5.10. B, C, E

Symptoms suspicious of a pulmonary embolism may include syncope, haemoptysis, chest pain (often pleuritic), breathlessness and fever. Physical signs of a pulmonary embolism include circulatory collapse, tachycardia, tachypnoea and pleural rub.

The chest x-ray may show linear shadows or a difference in density between the lung fields.

ECG changes may include right axis deviation, Q_3, T_3 and RSR$'$ pattern in leads V_1 and V_2 on a standard 12 lead ECG. In significant pulmonary embolism arterial blood gas tensions show reduced Pa_{CO_2} and Pa_{O_2}.

5.11. C

Asymptomatic bifasicular block, although it may be a precursor of complete heart block, probably does not necessitate a pacemaker unless Stokes–Adams attacks or other symptoms develop.

Second degree A–V block may respond well to atropine, or treatment of the underlying disorder—such as digitalis toxicity. Asymptomatic A–V block may be congenital, in any case chronic, and would not necessarily require the insertion of a pacemaker.

Sinus arrest may not only cause dizziness due to the dropped beats, but may also allow the development of nodal or ventricular escape if not treated.

Wolff-Parkinson–White syndrome is a disorder of accelerated conduction and responds well to β-blocking agents.

.12. In conversion of dysrhythmias by electrical shock therapy:

    A. The electric shock should occur on the upstroke of the T wave

    B. A light general anaesthetic is not necessary if d.c. conversion with synchronization is carried out

    C. a.c. shock is safer than d.c. shock

    D. Elective conversion needs no prior preparation of the patient

    E. Ventricular fibrillation responds well to cardioversion but may be caused during elective cardioversion of other dysrhythmias.

.13. Aortic stenosis

    A. Causes right ventricular hypertrophy due to increased afterload

    B. Is usually subvalvular

    C. May cause angina pectoris indistinguishable from that of ischaemic heart disease

    D. Causes ventricular dilatation early in its course

    E. Is often associated with atrial fibrillation.

.14. Idiopathic respiratory distress syndrome (RDS) of the newborn

    A. Is the second commonest cause of death amongst liveborn premature infants

    B. Is unlikely with a lecithin:sphingomyelin ratio of greater than 2:1 in the amniotic fluid

    C. Is more common in babies born to mothers with placenta praevia

    D. Often responds to negative end expiratory pressure

    E. Is due to a lack of surface tension-lowering substance, causing gross atelectasis.

Answers overleaf

5.12. E

In elective cardioversion, the shock is synchronized to occur 20 ms after the peak of the R wave; if the shock occurs on the upstroke of the T wave, ventricular tachycardia or fibrillation may occur.

a.c. shock is more likely to cause myocardial damage and is more likely to precipitate ventricular fibrillation than is d.c. shock.

Elective cardioversion should be preceded by oral anticoagulants for 4 weeks; digitalis should be withdrawn 24–48 hours prior to the procedure; and the patient should fast on the day of the procedure to decrease the risk of aspiration under the general anaesthetic. Short duration general anaesthesia is commonly indicated because the procedure is both painful and alarming.

5.13. C

Left ventricular hypertrophy, due to increased afterload, is the common feature of significant aortic stenosis.

Dilatation of the ventricle occurs late in the course of the disease and heralds terminal heart failure.

The obstruction is usually valvular, but may be subvalvular or supravalvular. Atrial fibrillation is often indicative of concurrent mitral valve disease and not due to the aortic valve disease.

5.14. B, C, E

Newborn RDS is the commonest cause of death in liveborn premature infants. It is rarely seen in term infants. Maternal factors contributing to the possibility of infant RDS include diabetes mellitus, toxaemia and placenta praevia because these are often associated with placental dysfunction and preterm births.

Treatment includes controlled oxygen therapy, environmental control in an incubator to decrease oxygen consumption, correction of acidosis and, in some cases, IPPV. Continuous positive airways pressure, with or without endotracheal intubation, is often useful.

For the following five questions (5.15–5.19) which show
investigations, indicate the cause(s) of hepatic cirrhosis in which
that investigation is useful:

- **A.** Haemochromatosis
- **B.** Primary biliary
- **C.** HB_S antigen positive
- **D.** Wilson's disease
- **E.** Alcoholic.

5.15. Mitochondrial antibodies
5.16. Serum caeruloplasm
5.17. Desferrioxamine test
5.18. Serum -antitrypsin$_{99}$
5.19. Liver scanning with Tc

**5.20. The following conditions may present as a pyrexia of
unknown (or undetermined) origin (PUO):**

- **A.** Brucellosis
- **B.** Scarlet fever
- **C.** Typhoid fever
- **D.** Enteric fever
- **E.** Dysentery.

5.21. Concerning rabies:

- **A.** Active immunization undertaken after a rabid bite is of no
practical value
- **B.** The usual incubation period is 1–2 months
- **C.** Virus growth is restricted to the CNS
- **D.** The virus can infect a wide range of host animals
- **E.** Ventilator therapy in ITU has significantly improved
prognosis.

Answers overleaf

5.15. B, C, E
5.16. D
5.17. A
5.18. None
5.19. All Correct

In cirrhosis the uptake of the isotope is reduced and patchy throughout the liver, with increased uptake by the spleen. There is no reliable difference on scanning between the different types of cirrhosis. The other tests are useful in the diagnosis of the cause of hepatic cirrhosis. In the established cirrhotic the most useful tests in monitoring hepatocellular function are prothrombin activity bilirubin levels and plasma albumin levels.

5.20. A, C, D

PUO implies an abscence of specific or localizing signs associated with persistent fever.

Scarlet fever produces a familiar rash leading to early diagnosis.

Dysentery may be mild and not show severe fever; if pyrexia is significant, it is associated with intestinal features, unlike enteric fever.

5.21. B, D

Because the incubation period is long, active immunity following a rabid bite may be life-saving. The virus in fact is widely disseminated throughout the body, especially in nervous tissue, but can multiply in other tissues (e.g. salivary gland, pancreas, muscle and connective tissue).

The fox is the main natural reservoir in Europe, rabid foxes transmitting the disease to wild, farm and domestic animals, especially dogs and cats. In South America the vampire bat is an important exotic host as it may develop latent infection.

The prognosis of established rabies is hopeless.

5.22. The following events predispose to an attack of subacute bacterial endocarditis (infective endocarditis):

 A. Acute rheumatic fever
 B. Dental surgery
 C. Patent ductus arteriosus
 D. Transient bacteraemia
 E. Vaccination with living attenuated organisms.

5.23. Usual associations with lepromatous leprosy are:

 A. Abundant 'acid fast' bacilli in the lesions
 B. Continuous bacteraemia
 C. Positive lepromin skin test
 D. Progressive disease with poor prognosis
 E. Slow development of symmetric skin lesions.

5.24. Stridor in infancy may be caused by:

 A. Bronchiolitis
 B. Acute tracheolaryngobronchitis
 C. Scurvy
 D. Acute epiglottitis
 E. Laryngomalacia.

Answers overleaf

5.22. A, B, C, D

Any factor which causes damage to the endothelium lining of the heart, heart valves or major vessels, or which promotes transient bacteraemia, increases the chance of acquiring subacute bacterial endocarditis. Vaccination with live vaccine does not give rise to SBE. In susceptible individuals undergoing dental surgery, prophylactic penicillin is indicated.

5.23. A, B, D, E

The progressive or lepromatous phase occurs when the individual shows high susceptibility to the disease. The lepromin test (analogous to the Mantoux reaction) is usually negative, whereas in the tuberculoid phase the lepromin test is always positive. All the other features are characteristic of lepromatous leprosy.

5.24. B, D, E

Bronchiolitis is a lower respiratory tract infection and rarely causes stridor. It is secondary to infection and the site of impact is the bronchiole; therefore, upper airway obstruction does not occur.

Acute tracheolaryngobronchitis leads to croup which is associated with inspiratory stridor.

Scurvy is caused by a vitamin C deficiency and does not cause stridor. Vitamin D deficiency and rickets may be associated with stridor.

Acute epiglottitis causes severe stridor, which may require emergency treatment with endotracheal intubation or tracheostomy if obstruction is severe enough.

Laryngomalacia (floppy larynx) causes mild stridor exacerbated by upper respiratory tract infection. It improves spontaneously at about one year of age.

5.25. Disseminated intravascular coagulopathy (DIC):

A. Responds well to heparin therapy in premature separation of the placenta

B. May occur in drug resistant *Plasmodium falciparum* malaria

C. May show a normal prothrombin and partial thromboplastin time

D. May complicate meningococcal septicaemia

E. May be precipitated by hypothermia.

5.26. Patients with liver disease presenting for anaesthesia are at an increased risk because:

A. Hepatic perfusion is reduced by about 25% even in light anaesthesia

B. Neurologic decompensation may occur with changes in Pa_{CO_2}

C. Postoperative analgesia may precipitate hepatic coma

D. They are much more sensitive to tubocurarine

E. They may have blood coagulation problems due to a lack of factors V, IX, X and decreased prothrombin levels.

Answers overleaf

5.25. B, C, D, E

Premature separation of the placenta as a cause of DIC is bes treated by Caesarian section. Heparin therapy only increases th blood loss in this condition.

Drug resistant *Plasmodium falciparum* malaria, hypothermia an meningococcal septicaemia are only a few of the disorders that ca lead to DIC. It is usually triggered either by entry of procoagulan materials into the circulation or by widespread endothelial cell damag with collagen exposure.

The usual screening tests of coagulation, prothrombin time an partial thromboplastin time may be normal following the acute phas of DIC. If the disorder becomes chronic, as in septicaemia haemolytic transfusion reaction, or promyelocytic leukaemia, th coagulation factor levels may become normal due to increase synthesis. Fibrinogen assays are more useful in assessment of chroni DIC.

5.26. A, B, C, E

Narcotic analgesics, diuretics, phenothiazines, most sedatives an pentazocine may precipitate hepatic coma. These patients ar commonly resistant to tubocurarine, partly due to increased globuli levels relative to albumin and partly due to reduced cholinesteras production. Tubocurarine is bound to plasma globulins.

Hepatic encephalopathy may be precipitated by hypoxia hypoglycaemia, hypovolaemia and hypotension. Particular attentio should be paid to prevention of these factors during anaesthesia.

Coagulation problems may be severe in patients with liver disease This may be treated with oral or intramuscular vitamin K and fres blood transfusion (for restoration of clotting factors).

5.27. A 47-year-old man presents with the complaint of sudden onset of double vision. This first occurred 3 months earlier and resolved overnight. However, a recent episode lasted 4 days. On further questioning he relates three or four episodes of dysphagia. His only other complaint is of occasional morning cough—he smokes 40–60 cigarettes per day. On examination he is noted to have a moderate bilateral ptosis and a weak grasp. Investigation of this patient would include:

A. EEG
B. Chest radiograph
C. Electromyography
D. Edrophonium test with 5 mg edrophonium intravenously
E. Serum electrolytes.

5.28. In the patient with a differential diagnosis of myasthenia gravis or myasthenic syndrome, the treatment may include:

A. Thoracic surgery, requiring increased doses of tubocurarine
B. Plasma exchange
C. Guanidine
D. Oral potassium supplements
E. IPPV.

Answers overleaf

5.27. B, C, E

Without further evidence of an intracranial lesion, an EEG is not indicated; even with symptoms and signs of an intracranial lesion an EEG would not be the most useful test.

A chest radiograph, both PA and lateral, would possibly yield vital information to the diagnosis—i.e. the presence of an enlarged thymus gland or of a parenchymal lung lesion.

Electromyography will also be of aid in the differentiation of the diagnosis. Both myasthenia gravis and myasthenic syndrome due to carcinoma of the bronchus can give the symptoms described; both show reduced response to electrical stimulation but the tetanic rate of stimulation gives an increased action potential in myasthenic syndrome.

The proper dose for the edrophonium test in an adult is 2 mg and even at this dose may cause muscle fasciculations, colic, salivation and diarrhoea in the test subject. Myasthenic syndrome is not appreciably improved by edrophonium.

Serum potassium levels may effect the degree of muscle weakness present; marked improvement may occur with correction of hypokalaemia.

5.28. B, C, D, E

Whether the patient has myasthenia gravis or myasthenic syndrome, he would be much more sensitive to any competitive neuromuscular blocking agent; 5 mg of tuborcurarine may cause prolonged apnoea. Both may require thoracic surgery, either a thymectomy in a myasthenia gravis patient, or for removal of the tumour in carcinoma of the bronchus. Both may require IPPV either postoperatively or due to inadequate respiratory function from muscle weakness.

Guanidine may improve muscle weakness in myasthenic syndrome because it facilitates acetylcholine release at motor nerve endings. Both conditions improve with correction of hypokalaemia.

Plasma exchange may be of benefit to both, but more so to the patient with myasthenia gravis. The exchange removes acetylcholine receptor antibodies.

5.29. A diabetic patient aged 28 years regulates his own insulin dosage, but usually needs about 80 units of soluble insulin per day in two or three doses. An acute attack of pyelitis develops which may precipitate:

    A. Respiratory arrest due to hypocapnoea
    B. Dehydration
    C. Hypokalaemia
    D. Aspiration of stomach contents
    E. Hypoglycaemia.

5.30. In typhoid fever:

    A. Chloramphenicol therapy increases relapse rate
    B. Chronic carriers often have gallbladder infection
    C. Leucopenia characteristically occurs
    D. Man is the sole natural reservoir
    E. TAB vaccination provides immunity.

5.31. Which of the following pituitary hormones have been shown to be produced by non-endocrine tumours?

    A. Melanocyte stimulating hormone (MSH)
    B. Gonadotrophins
    C. Serotonin
    D. Adreno corticotrophic hormone (ACTH)
    E. Histamine.

Answers overleaf

5.29. B, C, D

The patient is a moderately severe and unstable diabetic and with such an infection susceptible to diabetic keto-acidosis.

The respiratory drive is increased due to metabolic acidosis and is sustained in spite of hypocapnoea so that respiratory arrest does not occur.

The severely dehydrated patient may be hypovolaemic enough to develop thromboses and/or renal failure. Rehydration with normal saline with potassium supplements to replace the water and potassium lost due to the osmotic diuresis of hyperglycaemia should be instituted together with insulin therapy. Repeated potassium and blood sugar estimations are necessary for correction of the keto-acidosis.

The patient may be in precoma and is therefore at risk from aspiration of stomach contents. Hypoglycaemia is unlikely unless the enhanced diabetic state is overtreated. Continuous infusion of low dose insulin should obviate this complication.

5.30. A, B, C, D

TAB vaccine confers only a minimal protection in as much as it raises the number of organisms required for a minimum infective dose. Recovery from infection confers a much higher and more prolonged resistance, but even this is not complete. Chloramphenicol inhibits agglutinin formation and this may account for its paradoxical effect on the relapse rate.

Cholecystectomy ends the carrier state in about 85% of carriers, which emphasizes the important epidemiological role of gallbladder infection. Intermittent faecal excretion of *Salmonella typhi* may continue after clinical cure—convalescent excretors for a short period, temporary excretors for up to one year and chronic carriers well over one year. Excretors with no history of clinical infection are termed symptomless excretors.

5.31. A, B, D

ACTH, MSH, thyroid-stimulating hormone (TSH), cortisol releasing factor (CRF), prolactin, gonadotrophins, vasopressin and growth hormone have all been shown to be released by non-endocrine tumours. Serotonin and histamine are not pituitary hormones, although they may be involved in neurotransmission and may be secreted by non-endocrine tumours.

the following five questions (5.32–5.36) indicate those pituitary ɔrmones (A, B, C, D, E) which are most likely to be secreted by at tumour?

- **A.** ACTH
- **B.** MSH
- **C.** Gonadotrophin
- **D.** TSH
- **E.** Prolactin (in men).

32. Tumours of the lung
33. Teratomas
34. Chorionepithelioma
35. Thymus
36. Renal carcinoma

37. Differences between Cushing's disease and Cushing's syndrome include:

- **A.** A high plasma cortisol with retention of the diurnal rhythm in Cushing's disease
- **B.** Partial suppression with 2 mg dexamethasone in Cushing's syndrome, but not in Cushing's disease
- **C.** Hypokalaemic alkalosis is rare in Cushing's disease
- **D.** The urinary free cortisols per 24 hours are highest in adrenal tumours
- **E.** Metyrapone may decrease the 17 oxogenic steroids (OGS) in the urine in Cushings syndrome.

38. Adequate control of diabetic patients may be interfered with by:

- **A.** Obesity
- **B.** Formation of anti-insulin antibodies
- **C.** Pregnancy
- **D.** Intercurrent infection
- **E.** Change in renal threshold to glucose

Answers overleaf

5.32. A, B, E; 5.33. C; 5.34. D; 5.35. A, B; 5.36. E

Although other combinations are possible, these are the most likely combinations. By far the most common hormones secreted by non-endocrine tumours are ACTH and MSH. The tumours most frequently involved are those of the lung, thymus and pancreas. Prolactin release in men has been shown to be associated with both renal and bronchogenic carcinomas. Both non-endocrine testicular tumours and chorionepitheliomas have been shown to secrete TSH. Teratomas are often associated with the release of gonadotrophin.

5.37. C, E

Plasma cortisols are high in both Cushing's disease and syndrome, with very high levels in the syndrome when due to ectopic adrenocorticotrophic hormone (ACTH) and cortisol releasing factor (CRF); no diurnal rhythm is maintained in either condition. Cushing's disease (hypothalamic) may show a partial suppression, i.e. it suppresses with 2 mg dexamethasone, but not with 0.5 mg 6 hrly; neither adrenal tumours, ectopic ACTH, nor ectopic CRF as a cause of Cushing's syndrome will show suppression. The urinary cortisols (free) are highest with ectopic sources of ACTH and CRF, not with adrenal tumours or in Cushing's disease.

Metyrapone may give a fall in urinary 17 OGS. Its action is to block the final stage of production of cortisol, causing an accumulation of cortisol precursors (corticosteroids), 17 oxogenic steroids and metabolites of the corticosteroids.

Hypokalaemic alkalosis is the most important difference in that it rarely occurs with Cushing's disease. Its presence is usually indicative of Cushing's syndrome.

5.38. All correct

The obese patient has more difficulty maintaining adequate control of his blood sugar levels. In a very few patients, insulin therapy may be more difficult due to formation of anti-insulin antibodies to standard insulin preparations. Very pure insulins are available but are in short supply and expensive. The advantage of the very pure insulin is less fat atrophy and hypertrophy at the site of the injection and a lower dose (usually about 10% less) than of standard preparations.

Pregnancy and intercurrent infections both interfere with control of blood sugar levels.

The renal threshold to glucose may change in the course of the disease, due to nephropathy. The incidence of nephropathy increases with the duration of the disease; in some cases control must be maintained on serum blood sugar estimations alone as the urinary sugar level is no longer a reliable indicator.

5.39. Diabetic patients may develop peripheral neuropathies but, more importantly, autonomic neuropathies. In autonomic neuropathy:

    A. The parasympathetic supply to the heart is more affected than the sympathetic
    B. There is an increase in the incidence of sinus arrhythmia
    C. Postural hypotension may be present
    D. Loss of overshoot with a Valsalva manoeuvre indicates impairment of the sympathetic supply to the heart
    E. May be characterized by intermittent attacks of diarrhoea.

5.40. Longterm complications in diabetics include:

    A. Glaucoma
    B. Peripheral vascular disease
    C. Necrobiosis diabeticorum
    D. Meningioma
    E. Nephrotic syndrome.

5.41. In actinomycosis:

    A. Cervicofacial, pulmonary and abdominal disease occurs
    B. Colonies released in pus are called 'sulphur granules'
    C. Definitive diagnosis depends upon isolation of causative organism
    D. Limited epidemics occur in farming communities
    E. Multiple draining sinuses commonly occur.

5.42. Following rubella during early pregnancy, typically the child may be born with:

    A. Deafness
    B. Cataract
    C. Patent ductus arteriosus
    D. Vestibular disturbances
    E. Hydrocephaly.

Answers overleaf

5.39. A, C, D, E

The heart may be essentially denervated by the loss of both the sympathetic and parasympathetic supplies to the heart. Loss of parasympathetic function is more common, with a resultant tachycardia. With loss of the sympathetic supply denervation sensitivity to catecholamines may occur. There is loss of sinus arrhythmia with a fixed R–R interval on deep breathing, and a loss of overshoot with the Valsalva manoeuvre.

Postural hypotension, abnormal peristalsis of the oesophagus and intermittent diarrhoea, with loss of sphincter sensation, are not uncommon.

5.40. A, B, C, E

Vitreous haemorrhage in association with diabetic retinopathy may cause acute glaucoma in diabetics.

Systemic atherosclerosis is extraordinarily common in these patients and its severity depends upon the length of time from the onset of diabetes, not on the adequacy of the control of the blood sugar levels.

Necrobiosis diabeticorum is common in diabetics with peripheral vascular disease.

There is no known increase in the incidence of meningiomas in diabetics.

5.41. A, B, C, E

Actinomycosis results from endogenous infection secondary to local trauma, such as dental extraction or appendicectomy. The disease is sporadic with no evidence of transfer from animals or man to man. The greater prevalence of the disease in farming communities is probably the result of greater carriage of the organisms in rural communities where it is primarily a disease of farm animals. (A presumptive diagnosis may be made on typical histology.)

5.42. A, B, C

There is a 90% chance of fetal infection and 50% of children will show some abnormality if maternal infection has occurred during the first 8 weeks of pregnancy. Deafness, cataract and patent ductus are typical of the 'rubella syndrome'. Microcephaly is a known rubella-related abnormality. While a wide range of developmental problems have been attributed to maternal rubella, vestibular problems are rare.

5.43. A patient develops severe persistent headache with signs of
meningism and a scattered rash. A lumbar puncture is
performed. The CSF shows a lymphocyte pleocytosis, an
increase in protein but normal values for glucose and chloride.
Following the appearance of an icteric tinge in the sclera, the
patient improves for a while with regression of symptoms and
treatment is withheld pending CSF culture results. Within a
day or so, signs and symptoms recur but there is no
significant change in the CSF findings. The clinical course so
far is consistent with infection by:

A. Haemophilus influenzae
B. Leptospira canicola
C. Neisseria meningitidis
D. Pseudomonas aeruginosa
E. Streptococcus pneumoniae.

5.44. Hypercalcaemia may be associated with:

A. Carcinoma of the bronchus
B. Immobilization of a patient
C. Renal insufficiency
D. Hypoparathyroidism
E. Multiple myeloma.

Answers overleaf

5.43. B

Leptospiral infection commonly shows two phases. The more virulant strains, which cause serious infection, accentuate the early bacteraemic phase symptoms of fever, rigors, severe headache, episcleral injection and possibly jaundice and purpura. The CSF can be shown by dark ground microscopy to contain leptospira and these may be recovered on culture. The second 'immune phase' follows after a brief remission, with the recurrence of meningeal symptoms and CSF changes suggestive of benign aseptic meningitis. The CSF shows a moderate lymphocytic pleocytosis with raised protein and normal or slightly decreased glucose and chloride levels. Organisms are usually not demonstrable, but serial antibody studies show a significant rising titre. By contrast, the other organisms produce frank pyogenic meningitis.

5.44. A, B, C, E

Hypoparathyroidism is usually associated with a low serum calcium because the effect of parathyroid hormone is to increase serum calcium levels. In renal insufficiency the high serum calcium may respond well to parathyroidectomy—this is tertiary hyperparathyroidism. Immobilization for whatever the cause—prolonged illness, fracture, paraplegia, etc—will cause hypercalcaemia.

In multiple myeloma, hypercalcaemia is usually due to bony destruction and immobilization, and may lead to hypercalcaemia nephropathy.

Metastatic carcinoma affecting bone (as with primary tumours in the bronchus, breast, thyroid, kidney or prostate) may cause a raised plasma calcium. Occasionally hypercalcaemia may be abolished with local removal of the tumour and it is assumed that these tumours secrete a calcium-raising substance.

5.45. In grand mal epilepsy:

A. A specific 3 per second spike and wave pattern is present on the EEG
B. The patient often experiences an aura prior to attack
C. Most anticonvulsants should be withdrawn 24 hours prior to anaesthesia as they may interact with many anaesthetic agents
D. The seizure commonly starts in part of a limb and spreads in a more or less orderly fashion to become generalized
E. A period of flaccid coma usually follows an attack.

5.46. Management of the patient with sickle cell anaemia (SCA) includes:

A. Pre-oxygenation with 100% oxygen before induction of anaesthesia
B. Cooling blanket if the patient is pyrexial
C. Chest physiotherapy 4-hrly postoperatively
D. Exchange blood transfusion the day before operation
E. Giving 100% oxygen throughout the operation.

5.47. Pre-operative preparation of the patient with SCA would include:

A. Intravenous urea
B. 500–1000 ml 2.4% sodium bicarbonate intravenously
C. Immediate surgery as soon as the necessity is determined because the patient may have a sickle crisis if surgery is delayed
D. Systemic antibiotics
E. Blood transfusion before major surgery.

Answers overleaf

5.45. B, E

In grand mal epilepsy the patient experiences an aura before the attack; it may be stereotyped for the individual. It may be sensory or motor. Anticonvulsants should never be suddenly withdrawn. Many anticonvulsants induce liver enzymes and therefore may alter metabolism of anaesthetic agents, but it is far safer to maintain the patient on therapy with as little interruption as possible.

The period of flaccid coma following an attack may be accompanied by fixed, dilated pupils, absence of corneal and deep tendon reflexes and a positive Babinski reflex.

The 3 per second spike and wave pattern is characteristic of petit mal epilepsy. The seizure described in (D) is classically Jacksonian. Grand mal seizures are usually generalized from the outset.

5.46. A, C

Most centres agree that the proper peri-operative management of SCA patients includes pre-oxygenation with 100% oxygen, prevention of hypothermia, use of an increased FIO_2 during surgery (but not 100%), 4 hrly postoperative chest physiotherapy and controlled oxygen therapy by mask for 24 hours.

Exchange transfusion, when indicated, should be undertaken in stages during the week before surgery.

5.47. D, E

Delay of surgery will not prevent a sickle crisis, but immediate surgery without proper preparation of the patient may precipitate one. If at all possible the percentage of sickle cell haemoglobin should be lowered to less than 30% and the normal haemoglobin concentration raised to 10 g/dl by exchange blood transfusion prior to surgery.

Alkalinization with sodium bicarbonate does inhibit sickling *in vitro*, but has not been proven to do so *in vivo*; even if alkalinization was to be attempted, the given dosage is too great. The process of alkalinization is one of slow, careful titration and is of questionable benefit. This is also true for magnesium sulphate, urea, dextrans and cyanate, which also have anti-sickling claims. Many patients with SCA have recurrent chest infections and would probably benefit from prophylactic antibiotics.

5.48. Later complications that occur in the patient with SCA include:

A. Congestive cardiac failure
B. Liver abscess
C. Cholelithiasis
D. Pyelonephritis
E. Meningitis.

5.49. In a child with SCA, pretibial pain may be due to:

A. Osgood–Schlatter disease
B. Salmonella osteomyelitis
C. Aseptic infarct of bone
D. Ewing's sarcoma
E. Referred pain from the psoas major due to an appendix abscess.

5.50. An 18-year-old, tall, thin male presents in casualty complaining of breathlessness increasing over a 3 week period. There has been severe restriction of activity and intermittent severe chest pain in the last week. He states that his father died suddenly at an early age after the same symptoms. On examination he is noted to have decreased muscle tone and relatively long extremities. A marked kyphoscoliosis is present. Dullness to percussion and absence of breath sounds are noted over the left lower zone of the chest. A murmur is easily heard over the right upper sternum. A collapsing pulse is noted.

A. Diagnosis is usually confirmed by a chest x-ray
B. This constitutes a medical emergency
C. The chances of complete recovery are good (greater than 80%)
D. The probability of other members of the family being effected is almost non-existent
E. The patient may be treated conservatively with digoxin and observation.

Answers overleaf

5.48. All correct

Multiple splenic infarctions can lead to immunosuppression which will predispose the patient to a variety of infections. Local infarcts may become infected, as a liver infarct may become a liver abscess.

Congestive cardiac failure (CCF) may result from the high output state associated with chronic anaemia and the relative fluid overload found in these patients. CCF may be iatrogenic due to rapid transfusion during a full sickle crisis; therefore, central venous monitoring is advisable in this situation.

Due to the increased turnover of red cells, the incidence of gallstones is increased.

5.49. B, C

Aseptic infarct of bone is a quite common presentation in patients with sickle cell anaemia (SCA). This is often difficult to distinguish from osteomyelitis. SCA patients are immunosuppressed due to overload of the reticuloendothelial system with red cell fragments and in some cases from autosplenectomy resulting from multiple infarcts. Salmonella osteomyelitis is fairly common following aseptic infarct.

Osgood–Schlatter disease occurs in older children and is isolated over the tibial tuberosity.

Ewing's sarcoma is no more common in this group than in the general population.

Referred pain from the psoas does not occur in the tibia.

5.50. A, E

The patient has the hallmaks of Marfan's syndrome. Chest x-ray would show an aortic aneurysm and left lower lobe collapse. This does not constitute an emergency because the patient is stable. With the increasing symptoms surgery should be undertaken for repair (grafting) of the aneurysm urgently, but only with facilities for full cardiopulmonary bypass. The chances of complete recovery are less than 80%. Other members of the family should be investigated as the incidence of Marfan's syndrome is at least 3 per 200 000 with occasional sporadic mutants. As it is an autosomal dominant disorder, each sibling has a 50% chance of also being affected.

5.51. Ulcerative colitis

A. Characteristically has 'skip' lesions
B. May be associated with arthritis
C. At presentation should have three stool specimens examined for pathogens
D. May be treated with phosphate enema
E. May undergo malignant change, especially in the younger age group.

5.52. Primary tubercular foci commonly occur in the following situations:

A. Lower lobe of lung
B. Meninges
C. Skin
D. Terminal ileum
E. Tonsil.

5.53. Causes of segmental demyelination include:

A. Guillain-Barré syndrome
B. Alcoholic neuropathy
C. Porphyria
D. Carcinoma
E. Diphtheria neuropathy.

Answers overleaf

5.51. B, C, E

'Skip' lesions are associated with Crohn's disease of the colon. Ulcerative colitis may be associated with multiarticular arthritis, iritis, ulceration of the legs, pyoderma and anaemia. It may be treated with prednisolone enemas. All new presentations should have three stools examined to rule out amoebic colitis as the symptoms are the same. Malignant change is common in all patients with ulcerative colitis, but more so in the younger group of patients.

5.52. A, C, E

Tuberculous meningitis occurs secondarily to a focus elsewhere in the body. The other sites are all possible portals of entry of tubercle bacilli. However, primary infection of the ileum caused by *Moraxella bovis* is now rare since the introduction of pasteurization of milk although endogenous post-primary gut lesions still occur from swallowed tuberculous sputum. Primary lesions in the skin are an occupational hazard of laboratory workers, butchers, postmortem room attendants and laundry workers.

5.53. A, B, D

In Guillain–Barré syndrome sensitized lymphocytes destroy the Schwann cells causing segmental demyelination.

The mechanism of carcinomatous neuropathy is not known, but is presumed to be an immune response to the tumour cells. The sensitized lymphocytes then produce degeneration of the Schwann cells as in Guillain–Barré.

Alcoholic neuropathy is axonal—due probably to deficiency of B-complex vitamins causing either death of the cell bodies, or of the nerve (the most common example being foot drop), and segmental demyelination. Thiamine deficiency is more common in spirit drinkers.

Porphyria and diphtheria cause axonal degeneration. Porphyria can effect any part of the nervous system; diphtheria most commonly causes neuritis of cranial and cervical nerves.

5.54. In addition to joint abnormalities, other associations with rheumatoid arthritis are:

A. A normochromic, normocytic anaemia that responds well to iron therapy
B. Low plasma albumin
C. Ventilation perfusion inequalities
D. Coronary arteritis
E. Unusually fragile skin.

5.55. Prostaglandin F2^a administered in a therapeutic dose produces:

A. Water retention
B. Increased uterine contractility
C. Increased small bowel peristalsis
D. Dilatation of the bronchi
E. Elevation of the blood pressure.

5.56 Reduction of intracranial tension may effectively be achieved by:

A. Hyperventilation
B. Intravenous mannitol
C. Intravenous frusemide
D. Intravenous dexamethasone
E. Removal of CSF.

Answers overleaf

5.54. B, C, D, E

Rheumatoid arthritis is associated with a hypochromic, normocytic anaemia that is usually unresponsive to iron therapy. This may be potentiated by drug therapy with aspirin, phenylbutazone and steroids leading to gastrointestinal bleeding.

Plasma albumin levels may be low, which will alter the distribution of plasma bound drugs. It may also be associated with hypovolaemia.

The pericardium, myocardium and endocardium may all be affected by the disease. The degree of disability is difficult to assess as the patient may be greatly restricted by joint involvement. Coronary arteritis may show up as an ECG abnormality, especially of conduction.

5.55. B, C

Unlike other oxytocins, prostaglandins do not cause water retention. According to circumstances the prostaglandin can cause smooth muscle to constrict or relax. Because of constriction of the bronchi, caution is advised if prostaglandin F2^a use is contemplated in asthmatics. The relaxation of the smooth muscle of blood vessels would tend to lower blood pressure.

5.56. All correct

Hyperventilation with resultant hypocapnoea and vasoconstriction is beneficial in lowering intracranial tension. A Paco$_2$ of 4 kPa (30 mmHg) is probably the optimal level of hypocapnoea.

Intravenous diuretics are useful in the lowering of raised intracranial tension, with mannitol being the drug of choice, as it works directly as an osmotic diuretic. Frusemide is not as effective and may cause more electrolyte imbalance than mannitol.

Intravenous dexamethasone has been shown to be effective in the treatment of some causes of raised intracranial tension, especially tumours, and may be useful in preventing further rises in the tension.

Mechanical removal of CSF from the appropriate site is effective in lowering intracranial tension. Hydrocephalus is often successfully treated with *in situ* intraventricular drainage, with a shunt from the cerebral ventricle to the right atrium or the peritoneal cavity.

5.57. Causalgia:

   A. May be due to abnormal synapses at the site of nerve injury
   B. Results in efferent sympathetic impulses being circulated into sensory afferent fibers with ultimate thalamic interpretation of pain
   C. May cause release of bradykinin distally, producing a burning pain
   D. May be relieved by a stellate ganglion block
   E. May be relieved by a Bier's block with guanethidine

5.58. Patients with myocardial infarction:

   A. May present with pain in the left arm or wrist
   B. Require prophylactic diuretics to prevent pulmonary oedema
   C. Are a low risk when given local anaesthesia for hernia repair if well 3 months after infarction
   D. Have an increased incidence of peripheral vascular disease
   E. May develop ventricular aneurysm in the next year.

5.59. Iron deficiency anaemia:

   A. Is most commonly caused by dietary deficiency
   B. Has a hypochromic macrocytic picture
   C. Usually has high total iron binding capacity and a low serum iron level
   D. Is associated with a high reticulocyte count
   E. Is effectively treated with a 2 week course of oral iron tablets

Answers overleaf

5.57. All correct

Bradykinin release has been implicated in the burning pain of causalgia. When a limb is involved, effective forms of treatment include surgical sympathectomy, blocking of the sympathetic ganglia with local anaesthetic and Bier's block with guanethidine. The role of mood-altering drugs is also important, as emotional disturbances often exacerbate the condition.

5.58. A, D, E

Myocardial infarction pain may be felt in the left chest, jaw, arm or wrist. Although patients may need diuretics in the treatment of pulmonary oedema following a myocardial infarction, there is little evidence that their prophylactic use would decrease the morbidity associated with myocardial infarction, and may even be hazardous due to the electrolyte disturbance associated with their use. Coronary artery disease rarely occurs in isolation and is usually only part of a generalized vascular disease. Therefore, the incidence of peripheral vascular disease is higher in patients who have a myocardial infarction.

In the year following a myocardial infarction, the patient is at risk of developing a ventricular aneurysm.

Substituting local for general anaesthesia does not reduce the risks of further myocardial infarct, although it might ease the burden of responsibility on the anaesthetist. Non-urgent surgery should be postponed for at least 6 months.

5.59. A, C

Worldwide, iron deficiency anaemia is a dietary phenomenon. However, in western cultures, the most common cause is blood loss. Menstrual blood loss is the most common cause in women of reproductive age, and gastrointestinal tract loss in others.

There is a hypochromic microcytic picture on peripheral blood smear. Low serum iron levels occur in conjunction with an increased total iron binding capacity.

The reticulocyte count is low until the condition is treated and then it is increased.

The rate of rise of the haemoglobin level is generally 1 g/dl week on adequate treatment with oral iron. A further 2 to 3 weeks treatment for replenishment of iron stores is desirable.

5.60. Hereditary spherocytosis:

  A. Demonstrates sex-linked recessive inheritance
  B. Splenomegaly is usually present
  C. Causes haemolytic anaemia
  D. May lead to obstructive jaundice
  E. Requires splenectomy in infancy.

5.61. A 47-year-old Pakistani woman presents with a 6 week history of fever, loss of appetite and headache. On examination she has neck stiffness and a positive Kernig's sign. CSF results are as follows:
  WBC: 6000-lymphocytes 5400 mm³
          polymorphs   600 mm³
  RBC: 886 mm³
  Protein: 75 mg/dl
  Sugar: 0.2 mmol/l

  A. Appropriate further investigations include viral titres and CSF viral cultures
  B. The CSF results are compatible with pneumococcal meningitis
  C. The results are suggestive of a blood contamination
  D. The patient should be treated with penicillin and gentamicin
  E. Investigate further with a chest x-ray and tuberculin test.

5.62. Patients with cardiac disease:

  A. Should not be premedicated with opiates due to their myocardial depressant effect
  B. May need to come to theatre in a sitting position
  C. May be extremely sensitive to even small doses of intravenous barbiturate
  D. Should be intubated under light general anaesthesia without local analgesic sprays
  E. Which is complicated by pulmonary hypertension, respond well to cyclopropane as induction agent.

Answers overleaf

5.60. B, C, D

Inheritance is autosomal dominant mode. Splenomegaly is often present as a physical sign. Haemolysis occurs due to abnormality of the red cell wall.

Obstructive jaundice may occur in older children, or in adults, because of pigment gallstones causing biliary obstruction. The disease may occasionally present as obstructive jaundice.

Splenectomy in infancy is avoided due to the risk of infection following removal of the spleen when pneumococcal infections are the most common cause for concern; haemophilus influenzae has also been implicated.

5.61. E

Viral meningitis does not have a 6 week history. The results do not suggest a bacterial meningitis (polymorphs increased, sugar decreased, protein increased). There are not enough RBCs to suggest a traumatic tap.

This is most likely to be tuberculous meningitis, in which case a chest x-ray and tuberculin test are mandatory. Also penicillin and gentamicin would not be used for treatment of tuberculous meningitis.

5.62. B, C

Intramuscular morphine, or papaveretum, has been shown to be safe even in high doses in patients with minimal cardiac reserve. The anxiety and fear associated with surgery in the unpremedicated patient may induce overt cardiac failure.

When surgery is urgent, the patient may come to theatre in incipient or overt heart failure and may need to be transported and induced sitting up.

Patients with a low fixed cardiac output may collapse and die with even small doses of intravenous barbiturate. Cyclopropane may be the best induction agent for these patients except in the presence of pulmonary hypertension.

Incautious intubation of cardiac patients may be disastrous due to the high incidence of dysrhythmias and hypertension associated with intubation.

5.63. Cigarette smoking:

    A. May decrease the oxygen capacity of the blood by up to 15%
    B. Unless stopped at least one week before, may as well be continued until the time of surgery
    C. Is associated with an increased chance of peripheral vascular disease
    D. Carries no ill effects if the smoke is filtered to remove tar
    E. Decreases peripheral vascular resistance.

5.64. Diabetic ketoacidosis:

    A. Is not accompanied by a normal level of consciousness
    B. May be precipitated by infection
    C. Leads to salt depletion and potassium retention
    D. Should be treated with a short-acting insulin
    E. Is an absolute contraindication for anaesthesia unless the surgical condition is likely to be lethal while waiting treatment of the ketoacidosis.

5.65. Cystic fibrosis:

    A. Is autosomal dominantly inherited
    B. Usually presents in the neonatal period
    C. Has a good longterm prognosis if treated early
    D. Is an indication for intensive chest physiotherapy following general anaesthesia
    E. May present with malabsorption and failure to thrive in childhood.

Answers overleaf

5.63. A, C

Carboxyhaemoglobin levels may reach 10–15% in heavy smokers. Because the half-life of the HbCO dissociation is about 4 hours following the last cigarette, it is advisable to stop cigarettes 24 hours or more before surgery, especially in patients already at risk from hypoxia or undergoing any major procedure. The blood level of CO is higher in filtertip smokers than in non-filtertip smokers. The peripheral vascular resistance is increased in cigarette smokers as is the incidence of peripheral vascular disease.

5.64. B, D, E

Patients are often conscious if they present early in the episode of ketoacidosis. Any infection may precipitate ketoacidosis as insulin requirements are increased in spite of decreased carbohydrate intake. Osmotic diuresis, due to high blood sugar levels, occurs leading to sodium and potassium depletion which may be severe.

Short-acting insulin must be used in the treatment of ketoacidosis, either by continuous intravenous infusion or by hourly intramuscular injections. Long-acting insulin has a slow onset of action and may cause a late hypoglycaemia.

5.65. D, E

Cystic fibrosis is autosomal recessively inherited with 10–20% presenting during the neonatal period with meconium ileus.

The longterm prognosis is poor even with early diagnosis and treatment. In fact, early presentation may carry a worse prognosis as it may mean a more severe form of the disease. Survival beyond 25 years is uncommon.

Viscous secretions accumulate postoperatively in these patients. Vigorous preoperative and postoperative chest physiotherapy is needed to reduce the risk of postoperative chest infection.

5.66. Patients with cystic fibrosis:

    A. Respond well to bronchodilators
    B. Should be admitted for at least one week's physiotherapy and treatment prior to surgery
    C. Have abnormal sweat tests during childhood
    D. Are susceptible to recurrent chest infections
    E. Should have antibiotic cover for any anaesthetic.

5.67. A patient, 18 hours after eating a meal which featured tinned luncheon meat, develops severe stomach pains, vomiting and becomes prostrate. His general practitioner makes a tentative diagnosis of botulism:

    A. Blood cultures should be obtained for growth of *Clostridium botulinum*
    B. The appearance of cranial nerve paralysis is supportive of the diagnosis
    C. The administration of specific antitoxin is of marginal benefit once symptoms appear
    D. Hospitalization is mandatory
    E. Botulism is more common in the USA than in Western Europe.

5.68. Hypertension in childhood

    A. Is usually 'essential'
    B. Is usually present with coarctation of the aorta
    C. Does not require treatment
    D. May be secondary to renal disease
    E. Is treated with a salt-free diet.

Answers overleaf

5.66. B, C, D, E

The response of patients with cystic fibrosis to bronchodilators varies from showing slight improvement in peak flows and symptoms to showing no improvement. The typical pulmonary manifestation is bronchiectasis with alveolar destruction and fibrosis occurring later in the course of the disease. The most important aspects of treatment are physiotherapy and appropriate antibiotic therapy, as the bronchiectatic cavities are infected with a variety of organisms that change rapidly. Antibiotic prophylaxis for general anaesthesia should be given in relation to sputum culture and in conjunction with a week's pre-operative intensive chest physiotherapy to prepare for the procedure.

5.67. B, D, E

Botulism is a serious form of food poisoning caused by ingestion of food containing preformed exotoxins of the anaerobic sporebearer *Clostridium botulinum*. The source is inadequately sterilized preserved meats and vegetables, especially after home canning and bottling. Spores surviving the food processing later multiply with production of a potent neurotoxin. Symptoms appear 12–24 hours after the meal. Progressive cranial nerve paralysis develops with death occurring from respiratory paralysis or cardiac arrest. Administration of antitoxin may be life-saving.

Only 12 cases of the disease in Britain had been recorded until summer 1978 when an outbreak occurred in Birmingham involving 4 elderly people, two of whom died. The source of the toxin was thought to have been an imperfectly sealed can of North American salmon. Botulism is more common in USA, probably due to popularity of home bottling of vegetables.

5.68. B, D

Hypertension in childhood is rarely 'essential'; the most common cause of childhood hypertension is renal disease, although hypertension is an important sign in the diagnosis of coarctation of the aorta. Most children with hypertension require treatment. A salt-free diet is not an important part of its treatment as it is difficult to administer and children do not take well to this type of diet.

5.69. Red cell aplasia:

A. Usually presents in infancy
B. May be associated with systemic lupus erythematosis
C. Does not respond to corticosteroids
D. May be associated with a thymoma
E. May be associated with subsequent development of leukaemia.

5.70 In whooping cough

A. Most deaths occur in children under one year
B. The causative agent is *Bordatella pertusis*
C. Symptoms rarely persist more than 2 weeks
D. Is diagnosed from chest x-ray
E. Complications include lobar lung collapse.

5.71. A 6-week-old male infant presents with a 5 day history of vomiting and weight loss:

A. Jejunal atresia is a probable diagnosis
B. Urinary tract infection is a possible diagnosis
C. If a test feed confirms pyloric stenosis, immediate operation should be carried out
D. If the diagnosis is not obvious, the patient should be discharged home and reviewed in outpatients clinic in 10 days time
E. Barium enema is required.

Answers overleaf

5.69. B, D, E

Red cell aplasia rarely presents in infancy (the Blackfan–Diamond syndrome).

Red cell aplasia may be associated with many other haematologic disorders such as systemic lupus erythematosis, and also thymomas. Patients may subsequently develop leukaemia. Corticosteroids form an important part of the treatment of red cell aplasia.

5.70. A, B, E

Nearly all the mortality from whooping cough occurs in children under one year of age.

Bordatella pertussis is the causative agent.

Symptoms generally persist for many weeks and may be present for more than 2 months.

Chest x-ray may show collapse/consolidation, but does not give any specific diagnostic picture.

Complications include lobar collapse, which may lead to bronchiectasis if inadequately treated.

5.71. B

Jejunal atresia presents in the first day or so of life, as there is complete bowel obstruction.

A urinary tract infection can present in this manner and, if present at this stage, is often associated with congenital abnormalities of the renal tract.

Resuscitation with intravenous fluids is necessary if pyloric stenosis is the diagnosis. The operation should be performed during the day as it is not an emergency procedure.

Discharge home and review in 10 days time would likely have a high mortality as this could be an early pyloric stenosis or nearly any serious paediatric disorder. The patient should be admitted to hospital and investigated urgently.

A barium enema would not be indicated; the history is not typical of Hirschsprung's disease.

5.72. A 5-year-old child with patent ductus arteriosus:

   A. May have presented with failure to thrive
   B. Is inoperable if a loud pulmonary second sound and right ventricular hypertrophy on ECG are present
   C. Should have operation delayed until fully grown, if otherwise well
   D. On chest x-ray will show pulmonary oligaemia
   E. Should have a trial of medical closure with indomethacin.

5.73. A 3-week-old infant presents with failure to thrive and vomiting. The diagnosis may be:

   A. Gilbert's disease
   B. Congenital hypertrophic pyloric stenosis
   C. Coeliac disease
   D. Urinary tract infection
   E. Hydrocephalus.

5.74. Granuloma is a type of inflammatory reaction characteristic of:

   A. Tuberculosis
   B. Rheumatoid arthritis
   C. Regional ileitis
   D. Staphylococcal pyaemia
   E. Sarcoidosis.

Answers overleaf

5.72. A

Congenital heart disease can present as failure to thrive. In patent ductus arteriosus there is an increased metabolic rate due to left to right shunting through the lungs.

A loud pulmonary second sound indicates pulmonary hypertension and the ECG supports this. Generally the pulmonary hypertension is reversible, although cardiac catheter studies using 100% inspired oxygen will be necessary.

Operation to close the duct is recommended at 5 years of age as the morbidity and mortality associated with the operation is small and the chance of infective endocarditis in the untreated patient is high and carries considerable morbidity.

The chest x-ray in an uncomplicated patent ductus arteriosus shows plethora due to the left to right shunting.

Medical closure of the duct with indomethacin is successful only during the neonatal period.

5.73. B, D, E

Gilbert's disease, the commonest example of defective bilirubin transport, is a familial condition leading to hyperbilirubinaemia and presents with jaundice in a child that is not otherwise unduly ill.

Congenital hypertrophic pyloric stenosis also produces constipation and hypochloraemic alkalosis. It is easily corrected by Ramstedt's operation, after the child has been rehydrated and the alkalosis corrected.

Coelic disease does not occur until the child has been given gluten.

Urinary tract infections are a common cause of vomiting in neonates and may cause failure to thrive, as can hydrocephalus.

5.74. A, B, C, E

Granuloma occur in chronic inflammation, which share a common characteristic in that the inflammatory lesions take a nodular or tumour-like form. The term 'granuloma', though firmly established, is misleading. It implies a neoplasm of granulation tissue, but the tumour is simply a swelling. The granulation tissue is strikingly different from that of ordinary nonspecific infection (e.g. staphylococcal).

5.75. Severe haemolytic transfusion reactions are associated with:

A. IgM antibodies against non-ABO antigens
B. Bleeding at a previously dry operation site in the anaesthetized patient
C. Marked bradycardia
D. Marked haemoglobinaemia
E. Disseminated intravascular coagulopathy.

5.76. The following biochemical changes are likely to be found in a woman who has received an oral contraceptive containing oestrogen and progesterone for several months:

A. An increase in blood concentration of serum alkaline phosphatase
B. An increase in the blood concentration of protein-bound iodine
C. An increase in the blood concentration of free thyroxine
D. An increase in the blood concentration of fibrinogen
E. A reduction in the plasma concentration of cortisol.

5.77. Pulmonary embolism:

A. May be associated with a prominent 'a' wave in the jugular venous pulse.
B. Causes characteristic changes in the frontal axis ECG, including RBBB, T wave inversion in V_1 to V_3, 'p' pulmonale, development of an S wave in lead I and a Q wave with inverted T wave in lead III
C. May occur during surgical procedures undertaken in the sitting position
D. May be treated with fibrinolytic agents, such as streptokinase, to dissolve the clot
E. Can be accurately diagnosed on chest x-ray.

Answers overleaf

5.75. A, B, D, E

ABO incompatibility is the most common but IgM antibodies, against other blood group antigens, may cause a severe transfusion reaction.

The common symptoms and signs of the severe reaction—such as pain along the vein receiving the blood, flushing of the face, throbbing head, lumbar pain, chest constriction, tachycardia, hypotension, urticaria, peripheral circulatory collapse, rigors and pyrexia—are abolished by anaesthesia and the first sign of a problem may be bleeding from a previously dry operation site.

5.76. A, B, D

The amount of thyroid-binding globulin is elevated and as a result the free thyroxine is reduced. There is increase in plasma concentration of cortisol not a reduction. The T_4 concentration is likely to be raised, but not the free thyroxine level.

5.77. A, B, C, D

The prominent 'a' wave in the jugular venous pulse, following a pulmonary embolus, is due to decreased compliance of the right ventricle.

Air embolism may occur during neurosurgical procedures undertaken in the sitting position; most often during posterior fossa explorations. This can be diagnosed by a sudden drop in the expired CO_2 (pulmonary air embolism). Streptokinase may be effective in dissolving the clot in pulmonary embolism, but must be used with care as a massive haematoma may arise from an otherwise minor event such as an intramuscular injection.

Although chest X-ray may show differential blood flow it is of little use in the diagnosis of a pulmonary embolism in the first instance. It may however, show changes of pulmonary infarction if the patient survives the initial period. Embolism may be caused by any embolus, e.g. air, thrombus, pus, etc. All venous emboli reach the pulmonary circulation unless cardiac septal defects are present.

5.78. Convulsions during anaesthesia:

A. Occur only in those with a physical predisposition, such as children or epileptics
B. May be associated with 'malignant hyperpyrexia'
C. Are exacerbated by hypoxia and hypercarbia
D. May be a sign of septicaemia
E. Should be immediately treated with neuromuscular blockade and ventilation with 100% oxygen

5.79. In the management of chronic renal failure the following factors must be considered:

A. The prognosis following successful transplantation is far better than with longterm haemodialysis
B. The incidence of HBs antigen positive patients is increased in this group
C. The presence of a shunt or fistula gives easy access for intravenous fluid therapy or injection of drugs
D. High output cardiac failure may result from fistula formation
E. Although there are sufficient donor kidneys available, they do not have close enough HLA matching to be used in the patients awaiting transplantation.

5.80. Characteristically, syphilitic arteritis:

A. Is found in the aortic arch
B. Is found in the descending aorta
C. Causes intimal ulceration
D. Causes fibrous scarring
E. Produces aortic valve incompetence.

Answers overleaf

5.78. B, C, D, E

Convulsions under anaesthesia are rare. Classically, they were associated with di-ethylether. The evidence that all patients who have convulsions under anaesthesia have an epileptic tendency is inconclusive.

Sepsis leads to hypoxia and dehydration, which may precipitate a convulsion during anaesthesia.

Convulsion is part of the syndrome of 'malignant hyperpyrexia'. An epileptic discharge should be suppressed with anticonvulsants such as diazepam or thiopentone, but the safest immediate management lies in neuromuscular block.

5.79. B, D

The prognosis with successful transplantation and with longterm haemodialysis is about the same.

Due to the need for the repeated use of blood and blood products there is an increased incidence of HBs antigen positive patients.

As the lives of patients with chronic renal failure may literally depend on the presence of a functioning shunt or fistula, it should never be used for drug therapy or intravenous fluids. With an arm fistula, the resultant demand on the myocardium due to the large arteriovenous shunt may be unacceptably high. The low number of transplants in relation to the number of patients awaiting transplantation is due mainly to the inadequate supply of donor kidneys, although in theory the supply should be sufficient if permission to use most suitable kidneys could be obtained. With computerized records of tissue typing, a reasonable match can almost always be found for a donor kidney.

5.80. A, D, E

The abdominal aorta is rarely attacked in syphilis. The effects of syphilis are first noted in the tunica adventitia and spread inwards to the media where it destroys most of the elastic tissue. The intima is rarely affected.

5.81. In the normal cardiac cycle:

   A. The peak pressure in the pulmonary arterial system is approximately one-twentieth of that in the systemic arterial system.

   B. The first heart sound is caused by closure of the mitral and aortic valve

   C. Atrial contraction occurs in the early part of ventricular filling

   D. The stroke volume at rest is 60–100 mls

   E. Sympathetic stimulation increases the heart rate.

5.82. An immigrant child, recently returned from a holiday in his native country, develops fever and malaise. History-taking reveals that he has been in contact with diphtheria. Further examination results in a tentative diagnosis of diphtheria. Before initiating treatment with antitoxin it is a reasonable precaution to wait for:

   A. Bacteriological identification of *Corynebacterium diphtheriae.*

   B. Demonstration of toxigenicity

   C. First signs of cranial nerve palsies

   D. Formation of typical pseudomembrane

   E. Result of skin and ophthalmic tests for serum hypersensitivity.

Answers overleaf

5.81. D, E

The peak pressure in the pulmonary artery is approximately a quarter of that in the aorta. The first sound is caused by the closure of the mitral and tricuspid valves and the second sound by the aortic and pulmonary valves. Atrial contraction occurs in the late part of ventricular filling.

5.82. E

Any patient suspected of having diphtheria must be given antitoxin unless the skin and ophthalmic tests show serum hypersensitivity (tests take about 30 minutes). Positive reactors should first be desensitized. Prognosis is directly related to when antitoxin is first administered, and a delay of 24 or 48 hours—while waiting for the result of nasal and throat swab culture—may mean the loss of life.

5.83. A 2-year-old child presenting with cyanosis may have:

    A. Ebstein's anomaly
    B. Transposition of the great arteries
    C. Fallot's tetralogy
    D. Eisenmenger's syndrome
    E. Tricuspid atresia.

5.84. Ulceration of the bowel mucosa is characteristic of the following:

    A. Diverticulosis coli
    B. Coeliac disease
    C. Tuberculous enteritis
    D. Regional ileitis
    E. Typhoid fever.

5.85. A positive Schick test:

    A. Confirms a clinical attack of diphtheria
    B. Excludes the possibility of diphtheria
    C. Indicates the individual is a carrier
    D. Reveals susceptibility to diphtheria
    E. Shows that immunization is not required.

Answers overleaf

5.83. A, C, E

Patients with Eisenmenger's syndrome are usually symptom-free until late in the course of the condition. The reversed shunt (right to left) at atrial, ventricular or ductal level arises due to development of severe elevation of pulmonary vascular resistance.

Transposition presents in early infancy and is very unlikely to be alive untreated at 2 years of age.

5.84. C, D, E

Ulceration is not a characteristic feature of diverticulosis or coeliac disease. Mucosal ulceration is characteristic of the other conditions.

Crohn's disease is not readily distinguishable from chronic tuberculosis of the bowel. The typical typhoid bowel lesion is in the Peyer's patches which become inflamed and ulcerate. The ulcers may bleed or perforate, otherwise they heal with scarring.

5.85. D

Susceptibility to diphtheria is indicated by the appearance at 48 hours of a 1–5 cm inflamed and indurated area at the site of the intradermal injection of a standard skin–test–dose of diphtheria toxin provided the site injected with heat-inactivated (negative–control) toxin shows no reaction. A positive Schick test indicates the individual has insufficient circulating antitoxin to neutralize diphtheria toxin and requires to be immunized. Schick tests and throat cultures are usually done on contacts. Positive culture and positive Schick test indicates potential cases in need of treatment. Positive culture with negative Schick test indicates the carrier state. Negative culture with a negative Schick test shows the individual to be safe and not a public health risk.

6. SURGERY

6.1. Other congenital lesions associated with duodenal atresia include:

  A. Congenital heart disease
  B. Malrotation of the bowel
  C. Renal anomalies
  D. Congenital cataracts
  E. Deafness.

6.2. An abdominal x-ray of a neonate with persistent vomiting of bile-stained fluid shows two upper abdominal fluid levels with absence of air in the rest of the bowel. Likely diagnoses would be:

  A. Midgut volvulus
  B. Infantile pyloric stenosis
  C. Oesophageal atresia
  D. Annular pancreas
  E. Duodenal atresia.

6.3. An 18-hour-old male infant, with simian lines and facies of Down's syndrome, has persistent vomiting. The vomit is bile-stained. There is no abdominal distention and left to right peristalsis is visible. The initial stages of evaluation and management of this patient would include:

  A. Barium enema
  B. Abdominal radiograph
  C. Serum electrolytes
  D. Intravenous infusion
  E. Liver biopsy.

Answers overleaf

6.1. A, B, C

In addition to congenital heart disease, malrotation of the bowel and renal anomalies, other congenital lesions associated with duodenal atresia include oesophageal atresia, anorectal malformations, skeletal abnormalities and thirty per cent of these cases occur in Down's syndrome.

6.2. A, D, E

Infantile pyloric stenosis may present later in life, but in the neonate is not usually associated with bilious vomiting. Also only one upper abdominal air bubble would be seen.

Oesophageal atresia is unlikely without other symptoms (such as drooling) and, without an accompanying tracheo-oesophageal fistula, there would be no air in the bowel.

Midgut volvulus, annular pancreas and duodenal atresia are all causes of neonatal duodenal obstruction.

6.3. B, C, D

Duodenal obstruction is the presumptive diagnosis; duodenal atresia is often associated with Down's syndrome.

Barium enema and liver biopsy would not be helpful.

The persistently vomiting neonate will rapidly become dehydrated and may have severely deranged serum electrolytes. Intravenous therapy should be instituted to correct any electrolyte imbalance and to prevent further derangement of the body's biochemistry.

An abdominal x-ray is most useful in determining the level of obstruction.

6.4. Peri-operative management of a neonate undergoing surgery for correction of duodenal atresia would include:

A. Passage of a nasogastric tube
B. A barium meal 6 hours postoperatively to determine patency of the anastomosis
C. A transanastomatic tube for giving fluids and feeds
D. Rehydration
E. Chest x-ray, if not already done.

6.5. Treatment of squamous cell carcinoma of the face may include:

A. Radiotherapy
B. Wide excision of the lesion
C. Block dissection of the neck
D. Intravenous chemotherapy
E. Local chemotherapy such as 5-fluorouracil applied nightly for one month.

6.6 Predisposing factors to squamous cell carcinoma of the skin include:

A. Chronic ulceration
B. Syphilis
C. Dark-complexioned persons in tropical climates
D. Lupus vulgaris
E. Bowen's Disease.

Answers overleaf

6.4. A, C, D, E

Most children with duodenal atresia have some dehydration due to vomiting; this should be corrected pre-operatively.

The pre-operative decompression of the stomach is essential to prevent the aspiration of stomach contents at induction of anaesthesia. The decompression should continue postoperatively either through a nasogastric tube, or gastrostomy. The use of a transanastomatic tube is advocated by many surgeons for postoperative fluids and feeding. Fluid and electrolyte balance and nutrition should be maintained intravenously until full oral feeding is established.

A pre-operative chest film would be important in ruling out aspiration of vomit and in diagnosing any related cardiac abnormalities.

6.5. A, B, C, D

Depending on the site of the lesion, wide excision and/or radiotherapy are both useful. If regional lymph nodes are involved, block dissection may be useful in limiting lymphatic spread. Haematogenous spread of the disease occurs late. In far advanced squamous cell carcinoma, systemic chemotherapy may be useful in alleviating symptoms from metastases but cure is a rarity. Local chemotherapy with 5-fluorouracil would be of little use. Keratoses do respond but, once malignant changes have taken place, more vigorous therapy is indicated.

6.6. A, B, D, E

Squamous cell carcinoma of the skin is most common amongst fair-complexioned persons in tropical areas.

It may follow leukoplakia caused by syphilitic glossitis.

Bowen's disease is considered a pre-malignant lesion which may on rare occasions progress to squamous cell carcinoma. It resembles a plaque of psoriasis.

Lupus vulgaris may predispose to squamous cell carcinoma.

Chronic ulceration (Marjolin's ulcer) may progress to squamous cell carcinoma. It is by definition a malignant change in a scar, sinus tract, or ulcer, as in the case of chronic osteomyelitis sinuses, unhealed burns and chronic varicose ulcers.

6.7 A 3-year-old male of Nigerian parents is admitted from casualty with severe abdominal pain. The child has had previous episodes of similar pain that resolved after bedrest at home. He has not been followed at a child health clinic, but has been given iron tablets by the general practitioner. He also has a history of recurrent chest infections. On examination he has generalized abdominal tenderness and a pyrexia of 38.5°C. There is an area of marked tenderness over the right tibia. The initial investigations would include:

    A. Haemoglobin electrophoresis
    B. Abdominal and chest x-rays
    C. Red cell fragility testing with alkalinization
    D. Serum haemoglobin estimation
    E. Splenic arteriogram.

6.8. Malignant melanoma:

    A. Usually arises from a junctional nevus
    B. May arise from the pigmented layer of the retina
    C. Has a worse prognosis if it arises on the face
    D. Should be excised, followed by block dissection of the regional lymph nodes within 2 or 3 weeks
    E. Has a 50% 5-year survival rate when there is no lymph node involvement at the time of resection.

6.9. A 53-year-old, blue-eyed, sandy-complexioned civil engineer, who has been working in Saudi Arabia for 13 years, presents complaining of a 'skin rash' on his left cheek. The lesion has been present for 3–4 weeks. On examination a small (1.0 cm in diameter), conical, hard lesion is noted on the left cheek, just lateral to the angle of the mouth. There is a small area of ulceration in the centre of the lesion. The lesion is in an area of folliculitis; the patient explains that recurrent folliculitis has been a problem. Further investigation of this patient should include:

    A. Bacteriologic swabs of the area of folliculitis
    B. Biopsy of the small, hard conical lesion
    C. Chest x-ray
    D. Lymph node biopsy
    E. Liver biopsy.

Answers overleaf

6.7. B, D

Sickling in the splanchnic vessels may mimic many disorders. Patients with sickle cell anaemia (SCA) may present with abdominal, chest or bone pain. It is often difficult to distinguish between abdominal emergencies, such as acute appendicitis, and spanchnic sickling. The *initial* investigations should include serum haemoglobin estimation, chest x-ray and abdominal x-ray. A 'sickle-dex' should also be done; if this is positive, then haemoglobin electrophoresis should be done to determine the percentage of sickle haemoglobin.

6.8. A, B, D

Most malignant melanomas arise as malignant changes in a junctional nevus. Most are therefore cutaneous, but they may also be found on the mucous membrane of the anus, intestine, nose and mouth. They may also arise from the conjunctiva, the choroid and the pigmented layer of the retina. The prognosis is best when the lesion is located on the face. Adequately treated patients without lymph node involvement have a 5-year survival rate of about 75%; with regional lymph node involvement, the 5-year survival rate drops to 20%.

Adequate treatment includes the wide excision of the lesion with skin grafting; block dissection of the regional lymph nodes follows after 2 or 3 weeks. The delay is to allow any remaining malignant cells to be taken up by the nodes.

6.9. B, C

Bacteriologic swabs of folliculitis rarely give any useful information. Carriers of pathologic staphylococci may have recurrent folliculitis, but also usually have other lesions.

The small, hard, conical lesion is of greater concern. Its rapid progress could be an indication of a rapidly growing squamous cell carcinoma. Biopsy of the lesion need not be wide excision as in the case of malignant melanoma. Lymph node biopsy and liver biopsy are premature without definite histology. A chest x-ray, however, may show early metastases to the lung and will also serve as a baseline for future reference. Squamous cell carcinoma of the skin may rarely be a metastatic lesion from carcinoma of the lung.

6.10. The biopsy of the lesion in the previous case history was reported as being malignant. The type of malignancy is most likely to include:

    A. Malignant melanoma
    B. Keratoacanthoma
    C. Adenocarcinoma
    D. Squamous cell carcinoma
    E. Ephelides.

6.11. Postoperative pulmonary collapse:

    A. Has become relatively rare with modern surgical and anaesthetic techniques
    B. May be prevented by teaching the patient breathing exercises preoperatively
    C. May be aggravated by small doses of opiates
    D. Should be treated with a broad spectrum antibiotic
    E. Is most common following abdominal and thoracic surgery.

6.12. Dehiscence of an abdominal wound:

    A. Is more likely in the presence of chronic bronchitis
    B. Usually occurs on the fifth postoperaive day
    C. May be due to a wound haematoma
    D. Is often heralded by a pink fluid discharge from the wound
    E. Is rapidly followed by complete circulatory collapse of the patient.

Answers overleaf

6.10. D

Malignant melanoma is a possibility, but is unlikely with the given history and appearance.

Keratoacanthoma is a benign lesion that resembles squamous cell carcinoma. It may undergo degeneration to become squamous cell carcinoma.

Adenocarcinoma does not occur in this location and with this presentation.

Ephelides is a benign, extremely common lesion (juvenile freckles).

6.11. E

This complication is unfortunately still extremely common and is seen to some degree after almost every abdominal or thoracic procedure. Preoperative assessment and teaching of breathing exercises, in conjunction with postoperative physiotherapy, will help alleviate the situation but will not prevent it. Small doses of opiates are often useful as they diminish the pain of coughing and physiotherapy, but do not significantly dull the cough reflexes. Antibiotics should be given only if the sputum becomes infected, and then according to the sensitivity of the organism.

6.12. A, C, D

Factors predisposing to dehiscence of an abdominal wound include uraemia, cachexia, abdominal distention and chronic cough. It may be due to poor technique in suture of the wound or the use of low tensile strength suture material. Postoperative chest infections, with cough or ileus (causing distension of the bowel), may predispose to burst abdomen as do both infection of the wound or wound haematoma.

The dehiscence usually occurs around the tenth postoperative day and may be heralded by seepage of pink fluid from the wound. Following a cough, sneeze, or any strain, a loop of bowel or piece of omentum may then come through the suture line. The patient is usually in mortal fear at this stage and intramuscular opiates are useful in allaying anxiety. If the wound is covered with a sterile dressing soaked in saline and resutured, the prognosis is good for rapid, sound healing of the wound. The burst abdomen in itself should not cause circulatory collapse, unless the patient faints from the sudden appearance of a loop of bowel or piece of omentum.

6.13. Acute appendicitis:

   A. Is the commonest abdominal emergency
   B. Does not always necessitate emergency appendicectomy
   C. Has a higher morbidity and mortality during pregnancy
   D. Is easier to diagnose in the extremes of age
   E. May be mimicked by pleurisy.

6.14. Cleft lip and palate:

   A. Are usually associated with other congenital abnormalities
   B. Are to be repaired as urgent procedures because the infant cannot feed if complex cleft palate exists
   C. Were once termed hare-lip because the cleft is a median one
   D. Constitute major problems at intubation
   E. Are usually repaired separately.

Answers overleaf

6.13. A, B, C, E

It is commonest only in civilized communities, or in primitive peoples who change to western diet. Emergency appendicectomy is not the treatment of choice (1) in the moribund patient with peritonitis, (2) when the attack has resolved, (3) when an appendix mass has formed without evidence of peritonitis, or (4) when the circumstances surrounding the operation make it difficult, or impossible, (e.g. at sea). There is a higher morbidity and mortality during pregnancy due to the greater difficulty in diagnosis because of the displacement of the appendix. The diagnosis is more difficult in the extremes of age. Intrapleural pathology may give referred pain to the abdomen, especially in children.

6.14. E

They are not usually associated with other congenital abnormalities. The repair is undertaken between the third and the sixth month for cleft lip and at one year for cleft palate. If both conditions are present the lip is repaired at 8 weeks and the palate at one year. Cleft lip alone represents no feeding problems. The cleft palate interferes with the normal sucking mechanism, but the infant can feed normally from a spoon or by dropping milk into the mouth from a bottle with a large hole in the teat. The cleft rarely occurs in the midline. This may occur as failure of development of the philtrum from the fronto-nasal process, or in the cleft lower lip due to failure of the mandibular process to meet in the midline to form the lower jaw. The larynx and epiglottis are usually normal in these children. Although bilateral cleft lip and palate present the anaesthetist with unusual views of the oral cavity, no major problems with intubation are usually encountered.

6.15. Lung abscess may be associated with:

A. Dental extraction
B. Tuberculosis
C. Carcinoma of the lung
D. Metastatic cerebral abscess
E. Pulmonary metastases of carcinoma of the prostate.

6.16. Carcinoma of the breast:

A. May present as a fractured femur
B. Is the second commonest malignant disease of females in the UK
C. Shows a marked improvement in prognosis of the last 5 years
D. Is easily staged on clinical examination
E. May respond to androgenic steroids in older patients.

6.17. Carcinoma of the prostate:

A. Is usually transitional cell carcinoma
B. Is associated with osteolytic lesions and a raised serum acid phosphatase
C. Is usually discovered after it has spread beyond its capsule
D. May require adrenalectomy or hypophysectomy
E. May respond to castration.

Answers overleaf

6.15. A, B, C, D

Inhalation of a foreign body at the time of dental extraction is one of the commoner causes of lung abscess. Tuberculosis may cause lung abscess, but with modern therapy this complication is now rare.

Cerebral metastasis of the abscess is rare, but is also a recognized complication of lung abscess.

Although carcinoma of the lung may undergo degenerative change and become infected, or obstruct a bronchus, or bronchiole, causing a lung abscess, metastatic lesions to the lung occur only rarely.

Other causes of lung abscess include inhalation pneumonitis, infected cyst, infected pulmonary infarct secondary to blood-borne sepsis, and primary pulmonary infection such as pneumonia or bronchitis.

6.16. A

Pathologic fractures may be the presenting complaint in carcinoma of the breast because bony metastases occur rarely.

Carcinoma of the breast is the commonest malignant disease in females. No significant improvement in prognosis has occurred in the last 5 years. A high degree of clinical error (about 25%) exists in estimating between stage I and II.

Androgenic steroids may be useful in younger patients who have stage IV disease, or who have recurrences following mastectomy.

6.17. C, D, E

Histologically it is usually an adenocarcinoma, occasionally anaplastic. The bony lesions are usually osteosclerotic. Although a small adenocarcinoma may be found in a surgically removed prostate, most are discovered at an advanced stage. Although oestrogens, mainly stilboesterol, are the mainstay of treatment some refractory patients may respond to castration and/or adrenalectomy or hypophysectomy.

6.18. Carcinoma of the oesophagus:

    A. Is usually squamous cell carcinoma if it occurs at the lower end of the oesophagus

    B. Metastasises early to the liver and lungs

    C. May be resected if it occurs above the aortic arch

    D. May have symptoms relieved by the passing of a Mousseau--Barbin tube

    E. May be associated with Plummer–Vinson syndrome.

6.19. A 57-year-old man complains of pain in the calves and buttocks after walking 200 yards. Due to these symptoms he finds it difficult to carry out his job as a greengrocer. He also complains of cold legs and of impotence. On ECG he has significant Q waves in leads III and AVF. His management would include the following:

    A. Femoral arteriography

    B. Lumbar sympathectomy

    C. Fasting blood sugar

    D. Regular care by a chiropodist

    E. Femoral-popliteal bypass.

6.20. Internal haemorrhoids:

    A. Almost invariably bleed

    B. Have many predisposing factors, including portal hypertension

    C. May be complicated by anaemia

    D. Usually appear in the 2, 5 and 9 o'clock positions when the patient is in the lithotomy position.

    E. When treated surgically may cause serious postoperative haemorrhage.

Answers overleaf

16.18. D, E

Usually squamous cell tumours occur in the upper two thirds of the oesophagus, adenocarcinoma occurs in the lower third. Haematogenous spread to the liver and lungs occur late, local spread to the mediastinal structures occur early in the disease. Occurrence above the aortic arch is not usually resectable and may be treated by passing a Souttar's tube or a Mousseau–Barbin tube.

16.19. C, D

With buttock pain and impotence, the site of the lesion is probably terminal aorta and femoral arteriography would be hazardous. A translumbar aortogram would be necessary. With no rest pains, a lumbar sympathectomy may make claudication worse by diversion of blood to the skin. Atherosclerotic disease is frequently associated with diabetes mellitus, so a fasting blood sugar is indicated. Faulty foot care, such as trauma from nailcutting, may initiate gangrene; careful, professional chiropody is essential.

As the site of the lesion is proximal to the femoral artery, a femoral-popliteal bypass would not relieve this patient's symptoms.

6.20. A, B, C, E

Bleeding from internal haemorrhoids occurs primarily with defecation, often to the extent of causing anaemia.

Internal haemorrhoids are at the site of the systemic-portal anastomosis between the superior and inferior haemorrhoidal veins and therefore may form due to portal hypertension.

They appear at 3, 7 and 11 o'clock positions when the patient is in the lithotomy position.

Postoperative bleeding can require blood transfusion and re-exploration.

6.21. A 42-year-old woman complains of several episodes of pain across the lower sternum and radiating to the right scapula during the last 6 months. During one such episode she vomited several times and had dark urine for 24 hours. On examination she is noted to be moderately obese and to have yellow tinged sclera. Her management includes:

A. Intravenous morphine and bedrest for 3 weeks.
B. Plain abdominal x-ray
C. Liver function tests
D. Barium enema
E. Intravenous pyelogram.

6.22. A diverticulum of the bladder:

A. Is unimportant if congenital
B. Is caused when a bit of mucous lining is forced between the inner layer of hypertrophied muscle bundles
C. May cause ureteric obstruction
D. When complicated by an intradiverticular neoplasm, carries a good prognosis because tissue invasion is limited
E. May give rise to a vesical calculus.

Answers overleaf

6.21. B, C

Intravenous morphine has been reported to cause spasm of the Ampulla of Vater and exacerbates the symptoms of biliary colic. Although symptoms may be similar to those of coronary insufficiency, this patient is more likely to have gallbladder disease than coronary disease and therefore would not benefit from 3 weeks bedrest.

Plain abdominal x-ray reveals radio-opaque gallstones in 10% of cases. Liver function tests must be carried out in the presence of signs and symptoms of jaundice.

Barium enema would not be useful, but barium meal would be to exclude peptic ulcer and hiatus hernia.

Intravenous pyelogram would only be needed if there were symptoms other than those mentioned.

6.22. A, C, E

Congenital diverticulae are rare and unimportant because they empty normally with the bladder. The acquired (pulsion) diverticulum occurs when a bit of mucous lining is forced through all the muscle layers. This is usually due to high pressures (up to 100 cm H_2O) generated by the trabeculated bladder in endeavouring to force urine past an outlet obstruction.

As the diverticulum enlarges it may cause ureteric obstruction with hydronephrosis, hydroureter and, later, pyelonephritis and pyonephrosis. A neoplasm arising in a diverticulum is rare but, when it does, there is a poor prognosis because extravesical extension through the thin wall occurs readily.

Vesical calculi are present in 20% of the diverticulae due to stagnation and infection.

6.23. Hirschprung's disease:

A. Is usually not diagnosed until several weeks after birth
B. Is more common in females
C. Can be cured by excision of the aganglionic section
D. Can be diagnosed by biopsy of the anorectal wall
E. Can be differentiated from acquired megacolon by the absence of Auerbach's and Meissner's plexi in the wall of the colon.

Answers overleaf

6.23. C, D, E

Of all cases of Hirschprung's disease, 90% are diagnosed within the first 3 days of life. The neonate has constipation and abdominal distention, with loud borborygmi and visible peristalsis. It is much more common in males than females. Often it may be difficult to differentiate from acquired megacolon, in which case an anorectal biopsy will show the presence or absence of ganglia (Auerbach's plexus and Meissner's plexus). The only curative treatment for Hirschprung's disease is total resection of the aganglionic section. If possible the colon should be anastomosed to the anal canal. The child probably should not undergo resection until it weighs at least 8 kg. Interim treatment would include normal saline enemas and close observation for signs of increasing abdominal distention. Some authorities would advocate immediate transverse colostomy with definitive surgery delayed until the child weighs at least 14–15 kg.

**In the following six questions (6.24–6.29) indicate the relevant
clinical and radiological descriptions:**

    A. Occurs in the elderly
    B. May present as a pathologic fracture
    C. May appear as a soft tissue mass
    D. Area of bone destruction with ill-defined edges on x-ray
    E. May affect any bone with Paget's disease.

6.24. Osteosarcoma
6.25. Chondrosarcoma
6.26. Fibrosarcoma
6.27. Synovial sarcoma
6.28. Secondary neoplasm
6.29. Giant cell tumour

Answers overleaf

6.24. A, B, D, E

Osteosarcoma usually presents with pain and swelling and/or pathological fracture in the second or third decades, or in the elderly with Paget's disease. Ends of shafts of long bones, especially the femur, tibia or humerus, as well as any bone with Paget's disease, may be affected.

Although the tumour may go beyond the boundary of the bone to give a soft tissue shadow on x-ray, it does not present as a soft tissue mass. On x-ray the lesion appears as an area of destruction with ill-defined edges. Sunray spicules may be present. There may be pulmonary metastases which calcify. The 5-year survival rates vary, but are rarely over 15%.

6.25. D

Presents in the third or fourth decade and is locally invasive, giving rise to bloodborne metastases which are eventually fatal.

6.26. A, B, C, E

May present at any age and is of varying malignancy, giving rise to pulmonary metastases. The 5-year survival rate is about 30%.

6.27. A, C

The tumour presents as a soft tissue mass, most commonly associated with a joint, but it may arise in connective tissue, in muscle or subcutaneously. It may occur in any age group and appears on x-ray as a soft swelling, with or without spotty calcification. Regional lymph node involvement is not uncommon. Metastases occurs through the blood, lymphatics and also through the tissue planes of the limbs.

6.28. A, B, D

Two-thirds of secondary tumours of the bone arise from carcinoma of the breast or prostate.

6.29. B

Appears in the third or fourth decade as pain and swelling, with or without fracture and joint symptoms. It affects the epiphyseal region of the bone, expanding the bone and giving a soap bubble appearance on x-ray. Metastases are rare.

6.30. A 13-month-old infant is referred to an orthopaedic surgeon for assessment of possible congenital dislocation of the hip (CDH). In comparison with a neonate with suspected CDH:

A. The involved hip would be radiologically normal in the 13-month-old, but abnormal in the neonate
B. The involved hip in the older child would have full range of flexion, but will be limited in abduction with 90° of flexion
C. The acetabulum will appear unduly shallow in an x-ray of the older child
D. Von Rosen's sign will be positive in the older child
E. Examination of the hip of the older child will show a negative Trendelenberg's sign.

6.31. In the treatment of the older (over one year) child with CDH:

A. Closed manipulation is usually all that is needed as, once the hip is no longer dislocated, the ligaments will shorten enough to hold it in place
B. Unduly forceful closed manipulation may cause changes in the femoral head similar to those in Perthes' disease
C. Open reduction may be necessary due to fibrofatty tissue in the acetabulum
D. Six months immobilization in a hip spica is necessary
E. Pelvic osteotomy may be useful.

Answers overleaf

6.30. B, C, E

The radiograph of the hip of the neonate with CDH is normal, but in a child over 6 months old will be abnormal with:

1. Upward and outward displacement of the epiphysis of the femoral head.
2. A break in Shenton's line (a line along the inferior margin of the superior pubic ramus and the medial cortex of the femoral neck and shaft.
3. The capital femoral epiphysis is slow to develop and appears smaller on the affected side.
4. The superior lip of the acetabulum is also slow to develop and so appears unduly shallow.

Von Rosen's sign cannot be elicited in the older child as the hip will not abduct fully.

With a cooperative child a positive Trendelenberg's sign can be elicited at 13 months in unilateral disease. If the child has bilateral disease he would probably have developed the characteristic waddling gait of CDH.

6.31. B, C, D, E

Closed manipulation, with or without previous traction, may be successful in dislocating the femoral head, but undue force will jeopardize the blood supply to the femoral head. The acetabulum may fill with fibrofatty tissue so that closed manipulation is not successful. The presence of a fold of capsule or acetabular labrum may also interfere with closed reduction.

Whether open or closed reduction is required, the hip must be held in place with an appropriate form of splintage for a period of 6 months. Even after 6 months the results may not be satisfactory, which leads some surgeons to prefer surgical reconstruction of the hip in the form of pelvic osteotomy, a shelf operation, or intertrochanteric rotation osteotomy of the femur.

6.32. In congenital dislocation of the hip (CDH):

A. Treatment is easier in the neonate
B. There is a hereditary disposition for it
C. The occurrence is greater in females
D. The occurrence is lower with breech malposition of the fetus than with vertex presentation
E. The affected hip will not fully abduct at birth, except when dislocated.

6.33 Radiotherapy is a useful part of the treatment of:

A. Osteosarcoma
B. Chondrosarcoma
C. Secondary neoplasms of bone
D. Fibrosarcoma
E. Synovial sarcoma.

Answers overleaf

6.32. A, B, C

The ligaments at the hip are lax at birth in CDH. With correction of the dislocation and maintenance of the position, the ligaments will shorten over the next few months, and so the hip becomes stable and normal development can occur. This is usually all the treatment required if the CDH is treated in the neonatal period.

There are three predisposing factors to CDH:

1. Hereditary predisposition to joint laxity.
2. Female sex—possibly due to maternal 'relaxin' crossing the placenta and effecting the female fetus joints in the same way as it does the mother's.
3. Breech malposition of the fetus, possibly due to uterine pressure on the legs in the presence of lax ligaments causing dislocation.

The affected hip will abduct fully at birth only if the femoral head is not actually dislocated; it will abduct and dislocate with a characteristic 'clunk' (von Rosen's or Barlow's sign). When the femoral head is not in the acetabulum, the hip will not abduct; thus the distinction between the dislocated hip and the dislocatable hip.

6.33. A, C

The initial treatment of osteosarcoma is 9000 rads over 3 months to locally control the tumour. During the next 6 months most patients develop pulmonary secondaries from which they die, but without the mutilating surgery to remove the primary tumour. Those without the pulmonary secondaries at 6 months can then undergo amputation for removal of the primary.

Symptoms from secondary neoplasms of bone may be alleviated by radiotherapy to the affected area.

Chondrosarcoma, fibrosarcoma and synovial sarcoma are treated by resection. Chondrosarcoma is nearly always too large to be radiosensitive when diagnosed.

6.34. Neoplasms of the testis:

A. Are 99% malignant
B. Are most commonly teratomas
C. Are one of the commonest forms of cancer in the young male
D. Are preceded by trauma in 10% of cases
E. May present as lumbar pain.

6.35. Patients with head injuries:

A. Require early surgery for cerebrospinal fluid rhinorrhoea
B. May have a subdural haematoma due to rupture of the middle meningeal artery
C. Need urgent exploratory craniotomy if they are unconscious
D. Should be sedated with pethidine if restless
E. May have a 'lucid' period followed by unconsciousness and deepening coma.

6.36. Postoperative complications most commonly arising in the first 24 hours after surgery include:

A. Secondary haemorrhage
B. Reactionary haemorrhage
C. Aspiration pneumonia
D. Burst abdomen
E. Deep vein thrombosis

Answers overleaf

6.34. A, C, E

Of testicular tumours 99% are malignant, although they constitute only 1-2% of malignant tumours in the male. It is one of the commonest forms of cancer in the young male. The most common type is seminoma (40%), followed by teratomas (32%), combined seminoma and teratoma (14%), interstitial tumours (1.5%), lymphoma (7%), other tumours (5.5%).

Although about 10% of cases report history of trauma to be affected testicle, the trauma usually only calls attention to the enlargement and is not an initiating factor. Maldescent of the testicle is a predisposing factor. History of enlargement often extends to 4-6 months prior to advice being sought; indeed the enlarged testicle may be noted by an astute clinician when the patient presents complaining of abdominal or lumbar pain due to metastases. Prognosis depends on metastases and on histology.

6.35. E

CSF rhinorrhoea may be treated with barrier nursing and sulphadimidine while the patient's neurologic state is improving.

Middle meningeal artery rupture gives rise to extradural haematomas.

The patient may be unconscious due to conditions other than his head injury, such as diabetic coma, drug overdose, post-epileptic seizure, etc. Opiates given to head injuries not only depress respiration but also obscure valuable neurologic signs, such as pupillary reflexes and level of consciousness. A 'lucid' period, followed by headache and coma, is one presentation of an extradural haematoma.

6.36. B, C

Secondary haemorrhage, burst abdomen and deep vein thromboses usually occur after the first 24 hours. Vessels that have gone into spasm during the operation may relax and cause haemorrhage during the first 24 hours.

Aspiration pneumonia and asphyxia during the immediate postoperative period may occur due to depressed laryngeal reflexes after anaesthesia or after the administration of postoperative analgesia.

6.37. A slightly obese, 18-year-old female complains of severe abdominal pain for 8 hours. Other relevant history is of recent weight loss in spite of increased appetite and thirst. On examination she is found to have a rigid abdomen, a tachycardia of 120 beats/min and a respiratory rate of 35/min. It is noted that her breath smells rather sweet. No other relevant findings are present. BP is 130/70. Immediate management of this patient would include:

    A. Immediate laparoscopy to rule out ectopic pregnancy
    B. Serum urea and electrolytes, haemoglobin and blood surgar
    C. Intravenous pyelogram
    D. Intravenous infusion of IV saline while awaiting results of laboratory tests
    E. Erect and supine abdominal films.

6.38. In oesophageal atresia and tracheo-oesophageal fistula:

    A. Diagnosis is made by barium swallow
    B. Presentation is usually within the first 12 hours of life
    C. Management is nil by mouth and continuous suction to a tube at the site of the obstruction
    D. Aspiration pneumonia is a common complication
    E. Emergency operation is required as soon as the diagnosis is established.

Answers overleaf

6.37. B, D, E

Even with more evidence of ectopic pregnancy, it is rarely necessary to rush to theatre without adequate preparation of the patient. As the differential diagnosis is primarily between diabetic ketoacidosis and intra-abdominal pathology (appendicitis, volvulus, ectopic pregnancy), serum biochemistry should be done urgently and abdominal films done as an emergency. The tachypnoea and sweet-smelling breath indicate ketosis but not the diagnosis. Glycosuria and ketonuria should be tested for on admission.

With a stable BP any surgical procedure should be delayed if possible until the patient has been rehydrated and the ketosis corrected. Reassessment should then be carried out.

6.38. B, C, D

Barium swallow is extremely hazardous as the barium will end up in the bronchial tree. Presentation is nearly always within the first 12 hours of life with features such as frothy secretions from the mouth, collapse and cyanosis with bottle-feeding, pneumonia or Respiratory Distress Syndrome.

Suction, via a Refogle tube (double lumen) into the pouch of the oesophagus, is established.

Aspiration pneumonia may occur due to saliva or milk overflowing into the larynx or reflux of bile and gastric contents up the tracheo-oesophageal fistula.

If extremely ill, the child may need medical treatment, as above, plus antibiotics and ventilation to stabilize it before operation.

6.39. Coarctation of the aorta:

- **A.** If untreated may cause premature death due to intracranial haemorrhage
- **B.** Is best treated before the age of 5 years because permanent cardiac damage results if left longer
- **C.** May be pre-ductal or post-ductal
- **D.** When the clamps are released at surgery, a considerable increase in the proximal blood pressure occurs
- **E.** May require a jump graft during the corrective procedure if the coarctation is severe.

6.40. Ophthalmic complications of anaesthesia include thrombosis of the retinal artery which:

- **A.** Usually occurs in patients with pre-existing cardiovascular disease
- **B.** Causes blindness
- **C.** May be associated with compression of the eye by an anaesthetic mask
- **D.** May be part of a general syndrome due to hypoxia
- **E.** May be exacerbated by profound induced hypotension.

Answers overleaf

6.39. A, C, E

Premature death in the untreated patient occurs due to intracranial haemorrhage from the commonly associated berry aneurysm, heart failure, aortic rupture, or bacterial infection.

When preductal (proximal to the ductus arteriosus) it is usually associated with other cardiac abnormalities, and the children present at an early age in cardiac failure. Correction should be delayed until after 5 years of age unless cardiac failure demands early intervention.

With mild coarctation, which causes hypertension only with exercise, the collaterals may be insufficient to cope with the increased flow after clamping of the aorta. The proximal hypertension will then be quite high and may endanger the spinal cord and kidneys. In these patients a left atriofemoral bypass or temporary jump-graft will be needed to protect the spinal cord.

6.40. All correct

Retinal artery thrombosis is a relatively rare complication of anaesthesia and usually occurs in patients with pre-existing disease, such as temporal arteritis or polycythaemia. It may be induced by pressure on the eye, as from an anaesthetic mask, by hypotension or hypoxia.

For the following five questions (6.41–6.45) match the statement with the postoperative complication(s) it best describes:

    A. Deep vein thrombosis
    B. Bronchopneumonia
    C. Anaemia
    D. Secondary haemorrhage
    E. Staphylococcal enterocolitis.

6.41. Usually a late complication of surgery
6.42. Associated with pyrexia
6.43. May be associated with blood clot or infection
6.44. Best treated with erythromycin and neomycin
6.45. May occur following gastrectomy

Answers overleaf

6.41. C

Occurs most commonly following gastrectomy due to loss of intrinsic factor.

6.42. A, B, D, E

The patient with postoperative pyrexia should be examined carefully because the cause of pyrexia may be a wound or haematoma infection, staphylococcal enterocolitis, pelvic abscess, deep vein thrombosis, urinary tract infection, drug sensitivity, transfusion reaction, pulmonary collapse, bronchopneumonia, subphrenic abscess or diverse other conditions.

6.43. A, D

A blood clot or infection at the site of the wound may give rise to a secondary haemorrhage. A blood clot in the vein may be caused due to compression from a surrounding haematoma or infection around the vessel.

6.44. E

The cause of staphylococcal enterocolitis is usually an overgrowth of pathologic staphylococci following the administration of broad spectrum antibiotics. Good response follows the administration of erythromycin and oral neomycin. An alternative treatment is methycillin.

6.45. All correct

All the complications may follow gastrectomy. Deep vein thromboses, bronchopneumonia and secondary haemorrhage may follow any operation.

ANSWER SHEETS

Each question has five choices, A, B, C, D and E. Each choice may be true or false, and it is possible for all the five choices in any one question to be all true, or all false, or any intermediate combination.

Example:
1.10 Thyroytoxicosis is
       associated with

× A increasing weight
× B lethargy
× C low metabolic rate
✓ D rapid heart rate
× E peripheral vasoconstriction

In this example item D is true and items A, B, C and E false. Opposite each question number on the anser card are two rows of ovals, the upper marked T *(true)* and the lower marked F *(false)*. This question should be answered by making *black* marks on the appropriate answer card as follows:

	A	B	C	D	E
T	0	0	0	●	0
1.10 F	●	●	●	0	●

If you cannot decide whether a choice is true or false then do not mark either of the ovals for that choice.

Answer Sheets

	A	B	C	D	E		A	B	C	D	E
T 1.1	O	O	O	O	O	T 1.12	O	O	O	O	O
F	O	O	O	O	O	F	O	O	O	O	O
T 1.2	O	O	O	O	O	T 1.13	O	O	O	O	O
F	O	O	O	O	O	F	O	O	O	O	O
T 1.3	O	O	O	O	O	T 1.14	O	O	O	O	O
F	O	O	O	O	O	F	O	O	O	O	O
T 1.4	O	O	O	O	O	T 1.15	O	O	O	O	O
F	O	O	O	O	O	F	O	O	O	O	O
T 1.5	O	O	O	O	O	T 1.16	O	O	O	O	O
F	O	O	O	O	O	F	O	O	O	O	O
T 1.6	O	O	O	O	O	T 1.17	O	O	O	O	O
F	O	O	O	O	O	F	O	O	O	O	O
T 1.7	O	O	O	O	O	T 1.18	O	O	O	O	O
F	O	O	O	O	O	F	O	O	O	O	O
T 1.8	O	O	O	O	O	T 1.19	O	O	O	O	O
F	O	O	O	O	O	F	O	O	O	O	O
T 1.9	O	O	O	O	O	T 1.20	O	O	O	O	O
F	O	O	O	O	O	F	O	O	O	O	O
T 1.10	O	O	O	O	O	T 1.21	O	O	O	O	O
F	O	O	O	O	O	F	O	O	O	O	O
T 1.11	O	O	O	O	O	T 1.22	O	O	O	O	O
F	O	O	O	O	O	F	O	O	O	O	O

	A	B	C	D	E		A	B	C	D	E
T 1.23 F	0 0	0 0	0 0	0 0	0 0	T 1.34 F	0 0	0 0	0 0	0 0	0 0
T 1.24 F	0 0	0 0	0 0	0 0	0 0	T 1.35 F	0 0	0 0	0 0	0 0	0 0
T 1.25 F	0 0	0 0	0 0	0 0	0 0	T 1.36 F	0 0	0 0	0 0	0 0	0 0
T 1.26 F	0 0	0 0	0 0	0 0	0 0	T 1.37 F	0 0	0 0	0 0	0 0	0 0
T 1.27 F	0 0	0 0	0 0	0 0	0 0	T 1.38 F	0 0	0 0	0 0	0 0	0 0
T 1.28 F	0 0	0 0	0 0	0 0	0 0	T 1.39 F	0 0	0 0	0 0	0 0	0 0
T 1.29 F	0 0	0 0	0 0	0 0	0 0	T 1.40 F	0 0	0 0	0 0	0 0	0 0
T 1.30 F	0 0	0 0	0 0	0 0	0 0	T 1.41 F	0 0	0 0	0 0	0 0	0 0
T 1.31 F	0 0	0 0	0 0	0 0	0 0	T 1.42 F	0 0	0 0	0 0	0 0	0 0
T 1.32 F	0 0	0 0	0 0	0 0	0 0	T 1.43 F	0 0	0 0	0 0	0 0	0 0
T 1.33 F	0 0	0 0	0 0	0 0	0 0	T 1.44 F	0 0	0 0	0 0	0 0	0 0

	A	B	C	D	E		A	B	C	D	E
T 1.45	O	O	O	O	O	T 2.10	O	O	O	O	O
F	O	O	O	O	O	F	O	O	O	O	O
T 1.46	O	O	O	O	O	T 2.11	O	O	O	O	O
F	O	O	O	O	O	F	O	O	O	O	O
T 2.1	O	O	O	O	O	T 2.12	O	O	O	O	O
F	O	O	O	O	O	F	O	O	O	O	O
T 2.2	O	O	O	O	O	T 2.13	O	O	O	O	O
F	O	O	O	O	O	F	O	O	O	O	O
T 2.3	O	O	O	O	O	T 2.14	O	O	O	O	O
F	O	O	O	O	O	F	O	O	O	O	O
T 2.4	O	O	O	O	O	T 2.15	O	O	O	O	O
F	O	O	O	O	O	F	O	O	O	O	O
T 2.5	O	O	O	O	O	T 2.16	O	O	O	O	O
F	O	O	O	O	O	F	O	O	O	O	O
T 2.6	O	O	O	O	O	T 2.17	O	O	O	O	O
F	O	O	O	O	O	F	O	O	O	O	O
T 2.7	O	O	O	O	O	T 2.18	O	O	O	O	O
F	O	O	O	O	O	F	O	O	O	O	O
T 2.8	O	O	O	O	O	T 2.19	O	O	O	O	O
F	O	O	O	O	O	F	O	O	O	O	O
T 2.9	O	O	O	O	O	T 2.20	O	O	O	O	O
F	O	O	O	O	O	F	O	O	O	O	O

	A	B	C	D	E		A	B	C	D	E
T 2.21 F	0 0	0 0	0 0	0 0	0 0	T 2.32 F	0 0	0 0	0 0	0 0	0 0
T 2.22 F	0 0	0 0	0 0	0 0	0 0	T 2.33 F	0 0	0 0	0 0	0 0	0 0
T 2.23 F	0 0	0 0	0 0	0 0	0 0	T 2.34 F	0 0	0 0	0 0	0 0	0 0
T 2.24 F	0 0	0 0	0 0	0 0	0 0	T 2.35 F	0 0	0 0	0 0	0 0	0 0
T 2.25 F	0 0	0 0	0 0	0 0	0 0	T 2.36 F	0 0	0 0	0 0	0 0	0 0
T 2.26 F	0 0	0 0	0 0	0 0	0 0	T 2.37 F	0 0	0 0	0 0	0 0	0 0
T 2.27 F	0 0	0 0	0 0	0 0	0 0	T 2.38 F	0 0	0 0	0 0	0 0	0 0
T 2.28 F	0 0	0 0	0 0	0 0	0 0	T 2.39 F	0 0	0 0	0 0	0 0	0 0
T 2.29 F	0 0	0 0	0 0	0 0	0 0	T 2.40 F	0 0	0 0	0 0	0 0	0 0
T 2.30 F	0 0	0 0	0 0	0 0	0 0	T 2.41 F	0 0	0 0	0 0	0 0	0 0
T 2.31 F	0 0	0 0	0 0	0 0	0 0	T 2.42 F	0 0	0 0	0 0	0 0	0 0

Answer Sheets

	A	B	C	D	E		A	B	C	D	E
T	O	O	O	O	O	T	O	O	O	O	O
2.43						2.54					
F	O	O	O	O	O	F	O	O	O	O	O
T	O	O	O	O	O	T	O	O	O	O	O
2.44						2.55					
F	O	O	O	O	O	F	O	O	O	O	O
T	O	O	O	O	O	T	O	O	O	O	O
2.45						2.56					
F	O	O	O	O	O	F	O	O	O	O	O
T	O	O	O	O	O	T	O	O	O	O	O
2.46						2.57					
F	O	O	O	O	O	F	O	O	O	O	O
T	O	O	O	O	O	T	O	O	O	O	O
2.47						2.58					
F	O	O	O	O	O	F	O	O	O	O	O
T	O	O	O	O	O	T	O	O	O	O	O
2.48						2.59					
F	O	O	O	O	O	F	O	O	O	O	O
T	O	O	O	O	O	T	O	O	O	O	O
2.49						2.60					
F	O	O	O	O	O	F	O	O	O	O	O
T	O	O	O	O	O	T	O	O	O	O	O
2.50						2.61					
F	O	O	O	O	O	F	O	O	O	O	O
T	O	O	O	O	O	T	O	O	O	O	O
2.51						2.62					
F	O	O	O	O	O	F	O	O	O	O	O
T	O	O	O	O	O	T	O	O	O	O	O
2.52						2.63					
F	O	O	O	O	O	F	O	O	O	O	O
T	O	O	O	O	O	T	O	O	O	O	O
2.53						2.64					
F	O	O	O	O	O	F	O	O	O	O	O

Answer Sheets

	A	B	C	D	E		A	B	C	D	E
T	O	O	O	O	O	T	O	O	O	O	O
2.65						3.9					
F	O	O	O	O	O	F	O	O	O	O	O
T	O	O	O	O	O	T	O	O	O	O	O
2.66						3.10					
F	O	O	O	O	O	F	O	O	O	O	O
						T	O	O	O	O	O
						3.11					
						F	O	O	O	O	O
T	O	O	O	O	O	T	O	O	O	O	O
3.1						3.12					
F	O	O	O	O	O	F	O	O	O	O	O
T	O	O	O	O	O	T	O	O	O	O	O
3.2						3.13					
F	O	O	O	O	O	F	O	O	O	O	O
T	O	O	O	O	O	T	O	O	O	O	O
3.3						3.14					
F	O	O	O	O	O	F	O	O	O	O	O
T	O	O	O	O	O	T	O	O	O	O	O
3.4						3.15					
F	O	O	O	O	O	F	O	O	O	O	O
T	O	O	O	O	O	T	O	O	O	O	O
3.5						3.16					
F	O	O	O	O	O	F	O	O	O	O	O
T	O	O	O	O	O	T	O	O	O	O	O
3.6						3.17					
F	O	O	O	O	O	F	O	O	O	O	O
T	O	O	O	O	O	T	O	O	O	O	O
3.7						3.18					
F	O	O	O	O	O	F	O	O	O	O	O
T	O	O	O	O	O	T	O	O	O	O	O
3.8						3.19					
F	O	O	O	O	O	F	O	O	O	O	O

Answer Sheets

	A	B	C	D	E		A	B	C	D	E
T	0	0	0	0	0	T	0	0	0	0	0
3.20						3.31					
F	0	0	0	0	0	F	0	0	0	0	0
T	0	0	0	0	0	T	0	0	0	0	0
3.21						3.32					
F	0	0	0	0	0	F	0	0	0	0	0
T	0	0	0	0	0	T	0	0	0	0	0
3.22						3.33					
F	0	0	0	0	0	F	0	0	0	0	0
T	0	0	0	0	0	T	0	0	0	0	0
3.23						3.34					
F	0	0	0	0	0	F	0	0	0	0	0
T	0	0	0	0	0	T	0	0	0	0	0
3.24						3.35					
F	0	0	0	0	0	F	0	0	0	0	0
T	0	0	0	0	0	T	0	0	0	0	0
3.25						3.36					
F	0	0	0	0	0	F	0	0	0	0	0
T	0	0	0	0	0	T	0	0	0	0	0
3.26						3.37					
F	0	0	0	0	0	F	0	0	0	0	0
T	0	0	0	0	0	T	0	0	0	0	0
3.27						3.38					
F	0	0	0	0	0	F	0	0	0	0	0
T	0	0	0	0	0	T	0	0	0	0	0
3.28						3.39					
F	0	0	0	0	0	F	0	0	0	0	0
T	0	0	0	0	0	T	0	0	0	0	0
3.29						3.40					
F	0	0	0	0	0	F	0	0	0	0	0
T	0	0	0	0	0	T	0	0	0	0	0
3.30						3.41					
F	0	0	0	0	0	F	0	0	0	0	0

	A	B	C	D	E			A	B	C	D	E
T	0	0	0	0	0	T		0	0	0	0	0
3.42						4.8						
F	0	0	0	0	0	F		0	0	0	0	0
T	0	0	0	0	0	T		0	0	0	0	0
3.43						4.9						
F	0	0	0	0	0	F		0	0	0	0	0
T	0	0	0	0	0	T		0	0	0	0	0
3.44						4.10						
F	0	0	0	0	0	F		0	0	0	0	0
T	0	0	0	0	0	T		0	0	0	0	0
3.45						4.11						
F	0	0	0	0	0	F		0	0	0	0	0
T	0	0	0	0	0	T		0	0	0	0	0
4.1						4.12						
F	0	0	0	0	0	F		0	0	0	0	0
T	0	0	0	0	0	T		0	0	0	0	0
4.2						4.13						
F	0	0	0	0	0	F		0	0	0	0	0
T	0	0	0	0	0	T		0	0	0	0	0
4.3						4.14						
F	0	0	0	0	0	F		0	0	0	0	0
T	0	0	0	0	0	T		0	0	0	0	0
4.4						4.15						
F	0	0	0	0	0	F		0	0	0	0	0
T	0	0	0	0	0	T		0	0	0	0	0
4.5						4.16						
F	0	0	0	0	0	F		0	0	0	0	0
T	0	0	0	0	0	T		0	0	0	0	0
4.6						4.17						
F	0	0	0	0	0	F		0	0	0	0	0
T	0	0	0	0	0	T		0	0	0	0	0
4.7						4.18						
F	0	0	0	0	0	F		0	0	0	0	0

	A	B	C	D	E		A	B	C	D	E
T	O	O	O	O	O	T	O	O	O	O	O
4.19						5.1					
F	O	O	O	O	O	F	O	O	O	O	O
T	O	O	O	O	O	T	O	O	O	O	O
4.20						5.2					
F	O	O	O	O	O	F	O	O	O	O	O
T	O	O	O	O	O	T	O	O	O	O	O
4.21						5.3					
F	O	O	O	O	O	F	O	O	O	O	O
T	O	O	O	O	O	T	O	O	O	O	O
4.22						5.4					
F	O	O	O	O	O	F	O	O	O	O	O
T	O	O	O	O	O	T	O	O	O	O	O
4.23						5.5					
F	O	O	O	O	O	F	O	O	O	O	O
T	O	O	O	O	O	T	O	O	O	O	O
4.24						5.6					
F	O	O	O	O	O	F	O	O	O	O	O
T	O	O	O	O	O	T	O	O	O	O	O
4.25						5.7					
F	O	O	O	O	O	F	O	O	O	O	O
T	O	O	O	O	O	T	O	O	O	O	O
4.26						5.8					
F	O	O	O	O	O	F	O	O	O	O	O
T	O	O	O	O	O	T	O	O	O	O	O
4.27						5.9					
F	O	O	O	O	O	F	O	O	O	O	O
T	O	O	O	O	O	T	O	O	O	O	O
4.28						5.10					
F	O	O	O	O	O	F	O	O	O	O	O
T	O	O	O	O	O	T	O	O	O	O	O
4.29						5.11					
F	O	O	O	O	O	F	O	O	O	O	O

Answer Sheets

	A	B	C	D	E		A	B	C	D	E
T	0	0	0	0	0	T	0	0	0	0	0
5.12						5.23					
F	0	0	0	0	0	F	0	0	0	0	0
T	0	0	0	0	0	T	0	0	0	0	0
5.13						5.24					
F	0	0	0	0	0	F	0	0	0	0	0
T	0	0	0	0	0	T	0	0	0	0	0
5.14						5.25					
F	0	0	0	0	0	F	0	0	0	0	0
T	0	0	0	0	0	T	0	0	0	0	0
5.15						5.26					
F	0	0	0	0	0	F	0	0	0	0	0
T	0	0	0	0	0	T	0	0	0	0	0
5.16						5.27					
F	0	0	0	0	0	F	0	0	0	0	0
T	0	0	0	0	0	T	0	0	0	0	0
5.17						5.28					
F	0	0	0	0	0	F	0	0	0	0	0
T	0	0	0	0	0	T	0	0	0	0	0
5.18						5.29					
F	0	0	0	0	0	F	0	0	0	0	0
T	0	0	0	0	0	T	0	0	0	0	0
5.19						5.30					
F	0	0	0	0	0	F	0	0	0	0	0
T	0	0	0	0	0	T	0	0	0	0	0
5.20						5.31					
F	0	0	0	0	0	F	0	0	0	0	0
T	0	0	0	0	0	T	0	0	0	0	0
5.21						5.32					
F	0	0	0	0	0	F	0	0	0	0	0
T	0	0	0	0	0	T	0	0	0	0	0
5.22						5.33					
F	0	0	0	0	0	F	0	0	0	0	0

	A	B	C	D	E		A	B	C	D	E
T 5.34	O	O	O	O	O	T 5.45	O	O	O	O	O
F	O	O	O	O	O	F	O	O	O	O	O
T 5.35	O	O	O	O	O	T 5.46	O	O	O	O	O
F	O	O	O	O	O	F	O	O	O	O	O
T 5.36	O	O	O	O	O	T 5.47	O	O	O	O	O
F	O	O	O	O	O	F	O	O	O	O	O
T 5.37	O	O	O	O	O	T 5.48	O	O	O	O	O
F	O	O	O	O	O	F	O	O	O	O	O
T 5.38	O	O	O	O	O	T 5.49	O	O	O	O	O
F	O	O	O	O	O	F	O	O	O	O	O
T 5.39	O	O	O	O	O	T 5.50	O	O	O	O	O
F	O	O	O	O	O	F	O	O	O	O	O
T 5.40	O	O	O	O	O	T 5.51	O	O	O	O	O
F	O	O	O	O	O	F	O	O	O	O	O
T 5.41	O	O	O	O	O	T 5.52	O	O	O	O	O
F	O	O	O	O	O	F	O	O	O	O	O
T 5.42	O	O	O	O	O	T 5.53	O	O	O	O	O
F	O	O	O	O	O	F	O	O	O	O	O
T 5.43	O	O	O	O	O	T 5.54	O	O	O	O	O
F	O	O	O	O	O	F	O	O	O	O	O
T 5.44	O	O	O	O	O	T 5.55	O	O	O	O	O
F	O	O	O	O	O	F	O	O	O	O	O

	A	B	C	D	E			A	B	C	D	E
T	O	O	O	O	O		T	O	O	O	O	O
5.56							5.67					
F	O	O	O	O	O		F	O	O	O	O	O
T	O	O	O	O	O		T	O	O	O	O	O
5.57							5.68					
F	O	O	O	O	O		F	O	O	O	O	O
T	O	O	O	O	O		T	O	O	O	O	O
5.58							5.69					
F	O	O	O	O	O		F	O	O	O	O	O
T	O	O	O	O	O		T	O	O	O	O	O
5.59							5.70					
F	O	O	O	O	O		F	O	O	O	O	O
T	O	O	O	O	O		T	O	O	O	O	O
5.60							5.71					
F	O	O	O	O	O		F	O	O	O	O	O
T	O	O	O	O	O		T	O	O	O	O	O
5.61							5.72					
F	O	O	O	O	O		F	O	O	O	O	O
T	O	O	O	O	O		T	O	O	O	O	O
5.62							5.73					
F	O	O	O	O	O		F	O	O	O	O	O
T	O	O	O	O	O		T	O	O	O	O	O
5.63							5.74					
F	O	O	O	O	O		F	O	O	O	O	O
T	O	O	O	O	O		T	O	O	O	O	O
5.64							5.75					
F	O	O	O	O	O		F	O	O	O	O	O
T	O	O	O	O	O		T	O	O	O	O	O
5.65							5.76					
F	O	O	O	O	O		F	O	O	O	O	O
T	O	O	O	O	O		T	O	O	O	O	O
5.66							5.77					
F	O	O	O	O	O		F	O	O	O	O	O

Answer Sheets

	A	B	C	D	E		A	B	C	D	E
T 5.78	0	0	0	0	0	T 6.4	0	0	0	0	0
F	0	0	0	0	0	F	0	0	0	0	0
T 5.79	0	0	0	0	0	T 6.5	0	0	0	0	0
F	0	0	0	0	0	F	0	0	0	0	0
T 5.80	0	0	0	0	0	T 6.6	0	0	0	0	0
F	0	0	0	0	0	F	0	0	0	0	0
T 5.81	0	0	0	0	0	T 6.7	0	0	0	0	0
F	0	0	0	0	0	F	0	0	0	0	0
T 5.82	0	0	0	0	0	T 6.8	0	0	0	0	0
F	0	0	0	0	0	F	0	0	0	0	0
T 5.83	0	0	0	0	0	T 6.9	0	0	0	0	0
F	0	0	0	0	0	F	0	0	0	0	0
T 5.84	0	0	0	0	0	T 6.10	0	0	0	0	0
F	0	0	0	0	0	F	0	0	0	0	0
T 5.85	0	0	0	0	0	T 6.11	0	0	0	0	0
F	0	0	0	0	0	F	0	0	0	0	0
T 6.1	0	0	0	0	0	T 6.12	0	0	0	0	0
F	0	0	0	0	0	F	0	0	0	0	0
T 6.2	0	0	0	0	0	T 6.13	0	0	0	0	0
F	0	0	0	0	0	F	0	0	0	0	0
T 6.3	0	0	0	0	0	T 6.14	0	0	0	0	0
F	0	0	0	0	0	F	0	0	0	0	0

Answer Sheets

	A	B	C	D	E		A	B	C	D	E
6.15 T	O	O	O	O	O	6.26 T	O	O	O	O	O
6.15 F	O	O	O	O	O	6.26 F	O	O	O	O	O
6.16 T	O	O	O	O	O	6.27 T	O	O	O	O	O
6.16 F	O	O	O	O	O	6.27 F	O	O	O	O	O
6.17 T	O	O	O	O	O	6.28 T	O	O	O	O	O
6.17 F	O	O	O	O	O	6.28 F	O	O	O	O	O
6.18 T	O	O	O	O	O	6.29 T	O	O	O	O	O
6.18 F	O	O	O	O	O	6.29 F	O	O	O	O	O
6.19 T	O	O	O	O	O	6.30 T	O	O	O	O	O
6.19 F	O	O	O	O	O	6.30 F	O	O	O	O	O
6.20 T	O	O	O	O	O	6.31 T	O	O	O	O	O
6.20 F	O	O	O	O	O	6.31 F	O	O	O	O	O
6.21 T	O	O	O	O	O	6.32 T	O	O	O	O	O
6.21 F	O	O	O	O	O	6.32 F	O	O	O	O	O
6.22 T	O	O	O	O	O	6.33 T	O	O	O	O	O
6.22 F	O	O	O	O	O	6.33 F	O	O	O	O	O
6.23 T	O	O	O	O	O	6.34 T	O	O	O	O	O
6.23 F	O	O	O	O	O	6.34 F	O	O	O	O	O
6.24 T	O	O	O	O	O	6.35 T	O	O	O	O	O
6.24 F	O	O	O	O	O	6.35 F	O	O	O	O	O
6.25 T	O	O	O	O	O	6.36 T	O	O	O	O	O
6.25 F	O	O	O	O	O	6.36 F	O	O	O	O	O

Answer Sheets

	A	B	C	D	E		A	B	C	D	E
T	0	0	0	0	0	T	0	0	0	0	0
6.37						6.42					
F	0	0	0	0	0	F	0	0	0	0	0
T	0	0	0	0	0	T	0	0	0	0	0
6.38						6.43					
F	0	0	0	0	0	F	0	0	0	0	0
T	0	0	0	0	0	T	0	0	0	0	0
6.39						6.44					
F	0	0	0	0	0	F	0	0	0	0	0
T	0	0	0	0	0	T	0	0	0	0	0
6.40						6.45					
F	0	0	0	0	0	F	0	0	0	0	0
T	0	0	0	0	0						
6.41											
F	0	0	0	0	0						